# Anaesthesia in Midwifery

RUTH BEVIS  SRN, SCM, HVcert

*Anaesthetic Sister*
*Bristol Maternity Hospital*

BAILLIÈRE TINDALL · LONDON

Published by Baillière Tindall,
1 St Anne's Road, Eastbourne BN21 3UN

First published 1984

ISBN 0 7020 1023 5

Typeset by Herts Typesetting Services Ltd
Printed in Great Britain by J. W. Arrowsmith Ltd, Bristol

---

**British Library Cataloguing in Publication Data**

Bevis, Ruth
   Anaesthesia in midwifery.
   1. Anesthesia
   I. Title
   617'.96'024613      RD81

   ISBN 0-7020-1023-5

---

# Contents

Foreword ix

Preface xi

1 Background 1

2 Basic Anaesthetic Equipment 8

3 Drugs Used in Anaesthesia 26

4 Obstetric Physiology and Pharmacology 45

5 Requirements in Obstetric Anaesthesia 52

6 Typical Anaesthetic for Caesarean Section 56

7 Nursing Responsibilities 60

8 Problems in Obstetric Anaesthesia 83

9 Obstetric Analgesia 96

10 Drugs in Labour 105

11 Inhalational Analgesia 114

12 Epidural Analgesia 123

13 Other Regional Blocks 144

14 Resuscitation of the Newborn 151

Index 163

Obstetric care is neither completely effective nor wholly acceptable to the woman unless it is permeated with a sympathetic understanding . . . .

M. Myles

This book is dedicated to sympathetic midwives everywhere, and in particular to Shirley, without whose encouragement it would never have been written.

# Foreword

Midwifery is both an art and a science. Practical skills and clinical judgement in midwifery must stem from a knowledge of the sciences relevant to it. In this specialist book on anaesthesia and analgesia for midwives, Ruth Bevis, an experienced midwife, has integrated a sound theoretical basis with the clinical and practical aspects of the subject.

Some time ago Ruth Bevis identified the need for a teaching aid in anaesthesia in midwifery for midwives and students who were working in the operating theatre and labour wards of maternity units. In 1981 she produced a flip chart on the subject and was awarded second place in the Royal College of Midwives/Cow & Gate Open Scholarship. From this small beginning evolved the idea of a book covering the information needed by a midwife if she is to be an effective member of the team providing care to mothers who require anaesthesia. The related subjects of pain relief and resuscitation of the newborn have also been covered in making up this comprehensive text.

In keeping with the original idea, the author has included information about the equipment and techniques used in general anaesthesia and the role of the midwife during the critical period of administration of anaesthetics. If used widely, the book could make a valuable contribution to the reduction of maternal mortality from anaesthesia, a cause of death invariably cited in the triennial report of the Confidential Enquiries into Maternal Deaths.

Ruth Bevis has correctly identified the need for this book and in combining her experience as a labour ward sister with her skills in writing, she has achieved a publication which will no doubt prove to be a valuable textbook for students and a useful reference book for practising midwives. Whilst the advantages of a midwife writing for midwives are identifiable throughout the book, there is little doubt that its contents will also be of interest to others.

*R. M. Ashton*

# Preface

This book was born as a result of a brief to teach my midwifery colleagues enough about the basics of anaesthesia to enable them to assist the anaesthetist confidently and efficiently. Many people will assert that this is not a part of the midwife's role. As a committed midwife, my reply to this is that if we are to give our mothers and babies the best possible care throughout pregnancy, labour and the puerperium, we shall increasingly find ourselves caring for them before, during and after caesarean section, as modern obstetrics in the western world develops. With improved methods of detecting problems and earlier intervention, the increased incidence of caesarean section will undoubtedly persist, even if it does not rise to any extent. Anaesthetic assistance is readily available in many centres, but there will always be the occasion when it is not, particularly when cuts in services and personnel are inevitable, as at the time of writing. If the midwife suddenly finds herself assisting the anaesthetist, she will need a basic knowledge of the equipment, principles and problems involved if she is to assist him safely.

This book aims to give an introduction to this knowledge. It does not set out to rival the excellent texts already available, although it does question one basic assumption implied in the other books on the subject of obstetric anaesthesia and analgesia, and that is that the midwife will already have a working knowledge of the basics of anaesthesia and anaesthetic equipment. Many newly qualified midwives will have spent only two weeks observing in the operating theatre, and, although they will have received lectures on anaesthesia, they may recall very little of these. With the strict role definition current in the UK, many younger midwives will never have changed an oxygen cylinder. Their older colleagues, though proficient in such practical matters, may feel unhappy caring for the patient undergoing central venous and arterial pressure monitoring.

I have aimed to cover the same ground as the anaesthetist in his lectures to student midwives. Since much of this will be new material, I hope this book will prove a useful tool for the student.

I hope too that the section on regional blocks will be helpful. I have tried to differentiate clearly between epidural and spinal techniques. Spinal analgesia looks set to attain the popularity in the UK which it has been enjoying across the Atlantic. Many midwives are uncertain of the differences between the two types of block.

I do not wish to 'sell' epidural analgesia, and have tried to present a balanced view of its advantages and disadvantages. There is plenty of scope for debate and argument as to variations in management and technique and the likely outcome of such variations, but this book is not the place to discuss these. Anaesthetists and obstetricians will sometimes view epidural block differently, but we all need to bear in mind that our endeavours are aimed at providing care to both mother and baby. For some women it is the right form of analgesia, and for others it is not; this will probably continue to be so.

There are certain strands which I have endeavoured to weave into the text throughout. One is the necessity, despite high technology and the many pressures on the midwife, to see each patient as an individual and to treat her as her individual needs require. British obstetric practice has been under considerable scrutiny from the British public and its media in the recent past, and none of us has cause for complacency.

As concerted efforts are made to reduce maternal and perinatal morbidity and mortality figures, another strand, which I hope emerges clearly, is the recognition of the team effort required of us, together with our obstetric, paediatric and anaesthetic colleagues. At the same time, nothing, even in this 'age of the chip', quite replaces the good old-fashioned midwife – the 'with-woman'. Our medical colleagues are quite prepared to agree with O'Driscoll's assertion that the presence of a sympathetic midwife markedly reduces the need for analgesia. I hope that the strand indicating the importance of positive support, encouragement and reassurance of the woman before, during and after labour also shows itself clearly.

Since completion of the manuscript, approval for the use by UK midwives of trichloroethylene as an analgesic in labour has been withdrawn. Its use is nevertheless discussed in Chapter 11, since it will doubtless be helpful to midwives working elsewhere, particularly where facilities are less sophisticated.

Various references are made, throughout the book, to the United Kingdom Central Council for Nursing, Midwifery and Health Visiting (the UKCC). This body comes into being in June 1983, so that at the time of writing it does not actually exist, although it will have been established before this book is published. My thanks are due to Miss Anne Bent, Professional Officer (Midwifery) with the UKCC, for her help in dealing with this. I have quoted the rules of the Central Midwives Board for Scotland and Northern Ireland where these are different, as well as some of the relevant legislation. At this early stage I am unable to quote rule numbers or other references, and can only refer the reader to the appropriate handbooks and amendments as they become available.

My sincere thanks are due to my colleagues and friends, too numerous to mention individually, who have helped and encouraged me throughout the writing of this book. In particular I wish to thank Mrs Ann Bassett for her patience and her efficient typing of the manuscript; Dr David Wilkins, Consultant Anaesthetist, for allowing me free access to the word processor, which has been invaluable; Dr Brian Perriss, Consultant Anaesthetist, for his encouragement in the very early stages and his help with particular problems, which was very much appreciated; Dr Peter Fleming, Consultant Paediatrician, for his help with the subject of neonatal resuscitation; Paul Gowin and Chris Leslie for all their hard work with the illustrations; and Miss V. Ruth Bennett, Senior Midwife Teacher, for her critical appraisal of the manuscript.

*Ruth Bevis*

# 1 Background

'A mixture of powdered virgin's hair and dried ants' eggs in the milk of a red cow' sounds a most delectable recipe. This was a 17th century recommendation for the difficult labours of the day in a town in Massachusetts.

Although the ancient Chinese documented their use of opium, and other societies used hemp and mandrake for pain relief in labour, obstetric anaesthesia and analgesia only began to develop significantly in the middle of the last century. As anaesthetic techniques and anaesthetic agents were devised or discovered, obstetric anaesthesia and analgesia began to grow, almost, it seems, as a sideline, since only a few considered it necessary, desirable, or even permissible. Surgeons and obstetricians certainly thought pain a vital component of their endeavours and saw no good reason why it should be alleviated. The moralists of the mid-19th century upheld this view, and religious opposition also contributed to the slow acceptance of pain relief in labour.

It is interesting to look at some of the major events in the development of anaesthesia generally into the sophistication of the 1980s, and to consider these alongside developments in obstetric anaesthesia and analgesia.

## The 16th and 17th Centuries

Curare appears in documents of the 16th century, when the poison arrows of certain South American Indians were described. These poison arrows paralysed their victims without tainting the flesh, and were used for hunting. They were prepared from plant extracts, usually with considerable ceremony. It was Sir Walter Raleigh, returning from an exploration of the Amazon, who brought reports of this phenomenon back to the western world.

Another drug whose use was recorded in the 16th century, also in South America, was cocaine, the first known local anaesthetic agent. It was derived from the leaves of a plant found in Bolivia and Peru;

these leaves had been chewed by the locals for centuries. The stimulating effect of cocaine on the central nervous system produced a lessening of fatigue, allowing more work to be accomplished in the thin air of the Andes. The documentation of cocaine concerns its use among the Inca people, who commonly performed trephining operations (making burr-holes in the skull). This was facilitated by the surgeon chewing 'coca' leaves and allowing his saliva to drip onto the wound site, producing effective local anaesthesia.

Also in the 16th century, Cordus synthesized 'sweet oil of vitriol', or ether.

Intravenous injection was first described in the 1660s; the equipment used consisted of a bladder and a sharpened quill.

### The 18th Century

Oxygen was described in the 1770s by both Priestley and Scheele, who discovered it independently of one another.

At the turn of the 19th century, Davy, also famous for his miner's lamp, described the analgesic properties of nitrous oxide, or 'laughing gas', but did not pursue this promising property.

*The early 1800s.* In the 1840s came a spate of anaesthetic agents — ether, nitrous oxide again, and also chloroform. Although the advent of these agents was fraught with difficulties and setbacks, 1847 saw the first obstetric anaesthetic.

On January 19, 1847, Dr James Simpson, referred to by a contemporary as 'that vulgar male midwife', administered ether to a patient in obstructed labour. Later that same year he gave chloroform analgesia to a patient in labour. This technique gained respectability just a few years later, in 1853, when Queen Victoria received chloroform analgesia at the hand of Dr John Snow. Not one to revel in pregnancy or childbirth, Her Majesty pronounced herself well pleased with the labour preceding the birth of Prince Leopold, referring to the means of her relief as 'that blessed chloroform'. 'Chloroform à la reine' then became fashionable, and analgesia in obstetrics became a viable proposition, and was much sought after by the smart set of the day.

In the early 1800s came further documentation of arrow poisons. An eccentric Lancastrian squire, Charles Waterton, visited the wilds of Demerera. In his book, *'Wanderings in South America'*, he described the preparation of 'wourali', a word which later became curare.

Inevitably the first anaesthetic deaths were also recorded during these years.

Accounts of experiments in these early days make fascinating reading. They were usually conducted at the dinner table, often with hilarious consequences, and can hardly be described as clinical trials! There are various accounts of public demonstrations, notably the one staged by Horace Wells, a Connecticut dentist, in 1844. He had successfully extracted teeth painlessly, using nitrous oxide, but his public demonstration was a humiliating fiasco which delayed the acceptance of nitrous oxide for some twenty years.

Interestingly, at the same time as 'chloroform à la reine', came Alexander Wood with his hypodermic syringe and hollow needle.

*The late 1800s.* In 1880, McEwen described his technique of oral tracheal intubation.

Cocaine appears again in the mid-19th century, when it was added to many of the fashionable tonics of the day. Its local anaesthetic properties were appreciated by Karl Koller, a pupil of Sigmund Freud. He demonstrated its effect on the cornea, allowing surgery to be performed. Soon after this, the first recorded injection of local anaesthetic took place. Halsted, a Baltimore surgeon, showed its effectiveness by injecting it into his arm; unfortunately he subsequently became the first recorded cocaine addict in the western world. His addiction was treated with morphine, converting him to a morphine addict!

In 1885, Corning, a New York neurologist, had inadvertently injected cocaine into the sub-arachnoid space and produced 'spinal anaesthesia'.

Although an effective drug, cocaine suffered the disadvantages of being relatively toxic as well as addictive, so much effort was directed into the search for less toxic substances, leading to the eventual synthesis of procaine in 1904.

In 1895, Kirstein of Berlin introduced the first direct vision laryngoscope, while a few years later the first crude ventilator was used by Matas in thoracic surgery.

Interesting developments were also taking place on the obstetric front.

From St Petersburg came the first account of the use of nitrous oxide as an analgesic in obstetrics. This was in 1880, when Klikovitch used it together with oxygen. He was even able to demonstrate, with an intra-uterine catheter and a manometer, that it did not inhibit uterine action. At the turn of the century a nitrous oxide and oxygen apparatus was in use but not widely available, and interest in this particular area seems to have waned somewhat at this time.

## The 1900s

*The early 1900s.* Also at the turn of the century comes mention of the first intentional spinal anaesthetic. The first operative delivery under spinal anaesthesia was performed in Germany in 1901. The synthesis of procaine in 1904 was followed by many other local anaesthetic agents over the years.

'Twilight sleep' produced by an initial dose of morphine and scopolamine, followed by further injections of scopolamine, was introduced in 1902. Prolonged labour, a restless patient suffering from woefully inadequate analgesia, and an asphyxiated baby, were inevitable results, but 'twilight sleep' remained popular and in wide use until the 1930s. Its saving grace must have been the resulting amnesia, so relieving any distress of attendants and patient, at least in retrospect.

Topical application of local anaesthetic to the vulva and vagina in labour in 1910 was the forerunner of infiltration of the perineum with local anaesthetic, which was described by Gellhorn in 1927.

An important development arising from field surgery in World War I was that of endotracheal intubation in anaesthesia. Magill and Rowbotham were key figures in this development in the 1920s, and various items of intubation equipment still bear their names.

*The 1930s.* In the 1930s attention again focused on nitrous oxide, and Minnitt produced his well-known apparatus for self-administration by the patient of 'gas and air' in equal quantities. It is interesting that this apparently retrograde step should have been so successful, for 'gas and air' provided a very hypoxic form of analgesia. Indeed it has been suggested that the hypoxia was a component part of the analgesia — a horrifying thought today. However, by this time, the Central Midwives Board (CMB) established by the Midwives Act of 1902, was the body controlling the training and practice of midwives in England and Wales. The importance of Minnitt's apparatus was that it was approved by the CMB for use by midwives without medical supervision, following suitable instruction and training. Separate legislation was introduced for midwives in Scotland and Northern Ireland in 1930.

Inhalational analgesia for patients under the care of midwives thus became more widely available. The Lucy Baldwin apparatus, designed by a midwife, for the administration of nitrous oxide with oxygen rather than air became available at this time, but was never approved by the CMB for England and Wales, and could only be used by a medical practitioner or by a midwife under medical supervision. Midwives in Northern Ireland were permitted to use it by the CMB for Northern Ireland.

Grantly Dick-Read published *'Natural Childbirth'* in 1933. He postulated that fear, tension and pain were interrelated, and that alleviation of the first two factors removed the third.

In 1938, Crafoord's positive pressure respirator brought today's ventilators a step nearer.

Curare comes upon the scene again in the 1930s. Samples of the South American poison arrows were taken to an American pharmaceutical firm which was able to produce it in a purified form. It was then used, in 1934, to treat cases of tetanus, and in 1940, to prevent trauma in electro-convulsive therapy.

*The 1940s.* Trichloroethylene had first been used in anaesthesia in the USA in 1934, and in 1943 it was used in the UK as an analgesic in labour. Not until 1955 were the Emotril and Tecota Mark 6 inhalers approved by the CMB for use by midwives.

Pethidine was used in labour for the first time in 1940. It had first been produced in Germany in 1939.

As early as 1942 came reports of continuous caudal block by Hingson and Edwards in the USA.

Further developments in the psychological approach came from Velvouski in 1947 with the 'conditioned reflex' approach, which came to be known as psychoprophylaxis.

Muscle relaxants were introduced for general surgery when in 1942 Griffith and Johnson used curare, following its successful debut in the previous decade. This heralded a whole new era in anaesthesia, as patients now did not require such deep anaesthesia for the abolition of undesirable reflexes or for surgical access to the abdomen.

*The 1950s.* The CMB approved pethidine for use by midwives, and the narcotic antagonists came into use. Pethilorfan was hailed as the new wonder drug of obstetric analgesia, but failed to live up to expectations.

In 1956 halothane was introduced as an anaesthetic agent, and in 1959 methoxyflurane came into use.

*The 1960s.* Surprisingly recently, in 1962, Dr Tunstall of Aberdeen introduced nitrous oxide and oxygen pre-mixed in equal quantities in one cylinder.

The 'Entonox' apparatus for the administration of this nitrous oxide and oxygen mixture was approved by the CMB in 1965 for use by unsupervised midwives, following suitable training.

This was the end of the 'hypoxic analgesia' era, and all 'gas and air' apparatus had been withdrawn by 1970.

Paracervical block was popular in the USA and Scandinavia at this time, but was not widely used in Britain.

Lumbar epidural blockade began to come into its own in the UK at the end of the decade.

*The 1970s.* The last decade has seen general acceptance of active management of labour as a means of improving perinatal mortality figures. This has necessitated a sharp increase in hospital delivery rather than home confinement, and there has been a reluctance to classify a woman as low-risk as regards her pregnancy, except in retrospect. With 'active management' has necessarily come earlier and therefore more frequent intervention, and with acceleration of labour, reputedly more painful, has come the demand for more effective pain relief.

More open attitudes, a better informed public and high expectations of the medical profession and medical science also contribute to this demand.

*The 1980s.* The early 1980s have been characterized by the 'active birth' movement. A very vocal minority throughout the western world has been demanding, and will continue to demand, an increased flexibility in obstetric services, with freedom of choice for the consumer as to how and where she will deliver her baby. There is, of course, 'nothing new under the sun', and Michel Odent's theories and practices reflect those recorded over centuries of human history. Alongside ever-increasing technology and scientific research, his approach provides a fascinating contrast, and has much to commend it.

However, 'natural' methods used alone would see a return to natural wastage, and this is a matter of concern to all. Alongside the perinatal mortality and morbidity figures, and of equal importance and concern, are the maternal mortality and morbidity statistics. Anaesthesia features in this area as a contributory factor and sometimes as a sole cause, so that anaesthetists readily recognize obstetric anaesthesia as a challenging specialty.

## SUGGESTED FURTHER READING

Atkinson, R. S. Rushman, G. B. and Lee, A. J. (1977). *A Synopsis of Anaesthesia*, 8th edn. Bristol: John Wright.

Crawford, J. S. (1970). The anaesthetist's contribution to maternal mortality. *British Journal of Anaesthesia* 45: 70.

Plantevin, O. (1973) *Obstetric Anaesthesia and Analgesia*. London: Butterworth.

Thorwald, J. (1957). *The Century of the Surgeon*. London: Thames and Hudson.

# 2 Basic Anaesthetic Equipment

A selection of basic anaesthetic equipment is described in this chapter so as to give the midwife an understanding of the apparatus she may be handling if called upon to assist the anaesthetist.

## THE BOYLES MACHINE

The Boyles anaesthetic machine is a trolley designed to carry and deliver a controllable, metered flow of anaesthetic gases and vapours, and to provide the anaesthetist with a convenient and transportable working surface (Fig. 2.1). Boyles machines vary in style and size, some being relatively small and easy to move, while others may be required to carry a range of monitoring equipment and a ventilator.

### Gases

All Boyles machines carry oxygen and nitrous oxide; most carry carbon dioxide and some carry cyclopropane as well. In many centres, oxygen and nitrous oxide are now supplied from a central supply via a pipeline, but the anaesthetic machine always carries cylinders in case of a fault in the piped supply. Cyclopropane is sometimes used in general surgery, although it has the disadvantage of being explosive and expensive. Cyclopropane is only supplied in cylinders. Suction apparatus may be attached to the Boyles machine, and suction may be available from a piped supply. Each of the three basic gases, oxygen, nitrous oxide and carbon dioxide, has different chemical properties.

### Reducing Valves

Each gas is under different pressure in the cylinders, and a reducing valve on the Boyles machine modifies and regulates this pressure so that gas flow can then be accurately controlled.

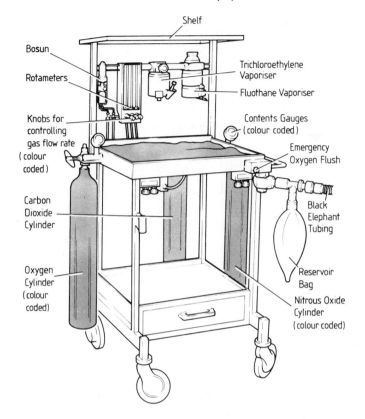

**Fig. 2.1** The Boyles machine. A typical anaesthetic machine.

*Colour Coding*

Gas cylinders are colour-coded as follows to comply with British Standards:

Oxygen —black cylinder with white 'shoulder'
Nitrous oxide —blue
'Entonox' —blue with blue/white 'shoulder'
Carbon dioxide —grey
Cyclopropane —orange

Gas cylinders cannot easily be connected to the wrong yoke because each cylinder and its corresponding yoke have a hole-and-pin system (Fig. 2.2). If cylinders are connected wrongly, it is only with some difficulty, and leakage of gas may result. The indicator dial for each gas is also colour-coded as above, providing a further safeguard.

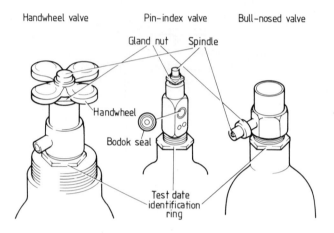

**Fig. 2.2** Types of cylinder head seen on medical gas cylinders. The 'pin-index' system is also shown.

*Bodok Seal*
Fitting round the gas inlet hole on the yoke, and between the faces of the cylinder and yoke, is a small rubber seal called a Bodok seal. This ensures a close fit and prevents leakage of gas. It will need to be replaced periodically.

Gases are checked before the Boyles machine is used, and cylinders should be used in strict rotation to avoid the situation where, for example, two almost empty cylinders are in position at the start of a procedure. To this end, clip-on labels — 'Full', 'In Use' and 'Empty' are available and should be used. The dial above the cylinder yoke gives a guide to the state of the cylinder contents. Gas flow is shown by flowmeters or rotameters (see Fig. 2.1). The rotameter is a vertical glass tube containing an aluminium bobbin which rises in relation to the gas flow. When gas is flowing, the bobbin should rotate. Gas flow is read from the top of the bobbin on the glass scale, which is marked in litres per minute.

Because medical gases are stored under pressure in the cylinders, and as each one liquefies at a different temperature, some will be stored as liquids. These are known as the liquefiable gases, and those in common use are nitrous oxide, carbon dioxide and cyclopropane. Because the cylinder contents will be partly liquid and partly gas, it is important to realize that the contents gauge will not indicate the amount remaining in the cylinder. The only reliable means of assessing the quantity remaining is to weigh the cylinder and its contents and to subtract the empty or 'tare' weight. Cylinders containing liquefiable gases have the 'tare' or empty weight marked on the valve or the shoulder of the cylinder.

Oxygen is referred to as a non-liquefiable gas because it is not liquefied by the application of pressure at room temperature. Because it remains stable in its gaseous state at room temperature, the contents gauge gives a reliable indication of the amount of gas remaining in the cylinder.

## Changing a Cylinder

Every Boyles machine should carry the appropriate cylinder key or spanner for opening and closing cylinders. When a cylinder is almost empty the following procedure should be adopted:

1. If the Boyles machine is in use, open the cylinder marked 'Full'. Check that gas flow is obtained before proceeding. If the Boyles machine is not in use, close all flowmeters.
2. Firmly close the empty cylinder, using the appropriate spanner or hand key on the spindle (see Fig. 2.2). Remove the cylinder from the machine and label it 'Empty' in accordance with hospital procedure.
3. Carefully remove the red seal from the new cylinder. (Do not push anything through the red seal into the pin index in order to break the seal.)
4. Before fitting the new cylinder, open it briefly using the cylinder key. This removes any foreign matter which would otherwise be blown into the system. Close the cylinder again.
5. Check the Bodok seal; if it appears worn it should be replaced.
6. Fit the cylinder, ensuring that the pins fit closely into the holes; replace the bracket which holds the cylinder in place and tighten the wing nut.
7. Use the cylinder key to open the cylinder again, in order to check

the integrity of the seal and the pressure within the cylinder. It should be opened slowly, and before use, it should be opened by two complete turns of the key.

8. No oil or grease is ever used on any gas cylinder or any part of the yokes, since this may cause a fire or an explosion.

## The 'Bosun'

Many Boyles machines have a warning system known as a 'Bosun', which is set off by any interruption to the flow of oxygen. This includes disconnection of the piped supply, or the emptying or closing of the oxygen cylinder while any other gases are flowing. Older models give an audible warning, while some have a red light which comes on to indicate any fault in the oxygen supply. Newer machines carry an 'oxygen failure warning device' which emits a whistle in the event of any failure of oxygen flow.

## Emergency Oxygen Flush

This is a system enabling the anaesthetist to fill the anaesthetic circuit quickly with oxygen. The patient's lungs can then be inflated using the black reservoir bag if necessary. The flush is operated by means of a knob which is usually on the front of the Boyles machine. (On the 'mini-Boyle', a small, easily transportable, anaesthetic machine, it is at the top, on the right side.)

## Volatile Agents

The volatile agents are used in conjunction with anaesthetic gases for maintenance of anaesthesia.

These volatile agents include halothane (or Fluothane), trichloroethylene (Trilene), methoxyflurane (Penthrane), enflurane (Ethrane), and ether. Each of these volatile agents is in liquid form at room temperature and, in order to be utilized, has to be vaporized and transported in a carrier gas. For anaesthesia, oxygen and nitrous oxide act as the carrier, but for obstetric analgesia, trichloroethylene and methoxyflurane are carried in air.

Each vaporizer on the Boyles machine is designed specifically for only one agent and must only be filled with the appropriate drug. Modern vaporizers are designed in such a way as to compensate for any outside factors which could influence rate of evaporation. These include the effects of change in temperature of the surrounding air and of the rate of carrier gas flow.

The vaporizer has a filling port at the side, and a small window where the level of fluid can be seen. The meniscus must always be visible, otherwise there may be doubt as to whether the apparatus is over-full or empty.

## Circuits
The anaesthetic circuit is the system of tubing and valves used to transport gases from the Boyles machine to the patient. Expired gases escape through an expiratory valve, and a ventilator may or may not be incorporated.

Circuits are classified under three headings — open, closed and semi-closed.

### Open Circuit
The open circuit is hardly ever used in the UK today. An example would be the use of ether on a Schimmelbusch mask.

### Closed Circuit
The closed circuit is one incorporating a carbon dioxide absorber; gases circulate and are then rebreathed. Fresh gas flow is thus much reduced, as is pollution of the theatre atmosphere. The usual means of absorbing carbon dioxide, which would otherwise accumulate, is a cannister of soda lime granules. Trichloroethylene cannot be used in a closed circuit as it reacts with soda lime to form toxic substances. The anaesthetist must therefore be informed if a patient in labour has received trichloroethylene (Trilene) analgesia prior to an anaesthetic, though this is unusual today. Closed circuits may be of the 'circle' type or of the 'to and fro' type. The latter is more cumbersome, since the soda lime cannister has to be positioned as near as possible to the patient.

### Semi-closed Circuit
The semi-closed circuit is the most commonly used type of circuit in the UK. It is one where a constant flow of fresh gas is required; it incorporates an expiratory valve through which exhaled gases go into the anti-pollution system or the atmosphere (Fig. 2.3).

*(a) The Magill circuit.* A typical semi-closed circuit is the Magill circuit, used for the anaesthetized patient who is breathing spontaneously. The Magill circuit consists of a face mask, angle piece, expiratory valve, a length of 'elephant' (black corrugated) tubing, and a reservoir bag.

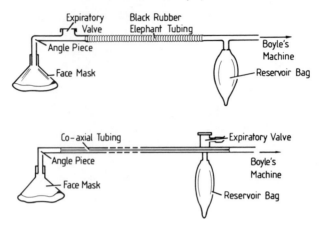

**Fig. 2.3** Semi-closed circuits: (a) the Magill circuit, (b) the Bain, or co-axial circuit.

*(b) The Bain circuit.* An alternative to the Magill circuit is the Bain or co-axial circuit. The Bain circuit consists of a length of narrow-bore tubing within a similar length of wider-bore tubing, hence the term co-axial. Fresh gas flows to the face mask or endotracheal tube via the inner tubing, and expired gases go directly into the outer tubing, usually to an anti-pollution scavenging system. The Bain circuit may be used with a ventilator, or for a spontaneously breathing patient.

**Face Masks**
A face mask is used for the patient who is breathing spontaneously. Various patterns exist and whichever type is preferred it must mould to the individual patient's facial contours so as to give an airtight fit around the nose and mouth.

Face masks are commonly made of black rubber, but for use in obstetrics where pre-oxygenation of 3–5 minutes is often given prior to induction of anaesthesia, the Ambu mask may be preferred. The Ambu mask (Fig. 2.4) consists of a transparent perspex face-piece surrounded by an inflatable, detachable black rubber rim.

Patients tend to object less to this type of mask; it is lighter, and fewer patients complain of feeling claustrophobic. If this mask is used throughout an anaesthetic, the patient's colour can be more easily observed, and, more important, any vomitus or secretions can be seen

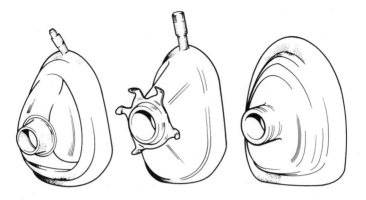

**Fig. 2.4** Face masks — from left to right: The Ambu mask, made of clear perspex with a detachable, black rubber rim; the BOC mask; the McKesson mask.

and removed. It is easily cleaned because of its detachable rim, which can be replaced whenever necessary.

Another type of face mask is the BOC mask. This mask is useful because, as well as having an inflatable rim, the mask itself can be moulded to fit the individual patient, being made of stiff black rubber. It is available in various sizes. The Everseal and McKesson patterns may also be used.

The face mask is used with an angle piece which connects the mask to the circuit tubing. The angle piece has a male and a female taper.

## EQUIPMENT REQUIRED FOR ENDOTRACHEAL INTUBATION

Intubation of the trachea with a cuffed endotracheal tube is generally considered to be a vital part of safe obstetric anaesthesia. The equipment required includes:

A laryngoscope
A cuffed oral endotracheal tube
Lubricant
A connector
A catheter mount
A 10 ml syringe to inflate the cuff
A pair of artery forceps to clamp the pilot tubing of the cuff

Tape to secure the tube in position.

An introducer may or may not be required.

### Laryngoscopes

Two types of laryngoscope blade are in common use for the purpose of intubation. Each of these types, plus various others which are available, come with either the American 'hook-on' fitting or the screw type fitting. The laryngoscope handle also comes in either of these designs. The handle carries the batteries providing the light source.

*The Macintosh laryngoscope.* This has a blade with a curved design (Fig. 2.5). The tip of the blade is passed anterior to the epiglottis and lifts the base of the tongue. The epiglottis is attached to the base of the tongue and is indirectly reflected to reveal the larynx.

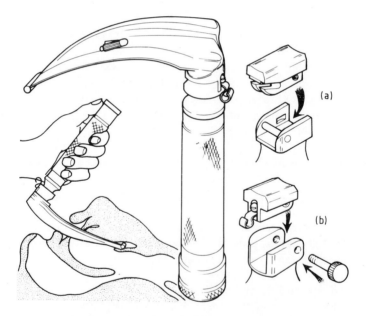

**Fig. 2.5** The Macintosh laryngoscope and its mode of action. Note how the blade slides over the tongue so that the blade tip lies between the epiglottis and the base of the tongue. Close-ups (a) and (b) show the American 'hook-on' fitting and the standard screw type fitting respectively.

*The Magill laryngoscope.* The blade is straight and is designed to sit posterior to the epiglottis and lift it directly to show the larynx (Fig. 2.6).

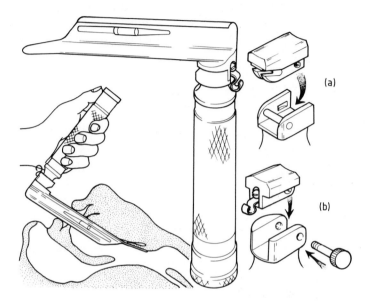

(a)

(b)

**Fig. 2.6** The Magill laryngoscope and its mode of action. The blade slips over the tongue and the epiglottis. (a) The American 'hook-on' fitting, (b) the standard screw type fitting.

The anaesthetist holds the laryngoscope in his left hand during intubation of the trachea. It is not used with a lever action, but the whole blade is gently lifted in a vertical plane. Even so, the upper teeth may be damaged during laryngoscopy, and the anaesthetist must thus be aware of the presence of any dental bridges, crowns or loose teeth.

### Endotracheal Tubes
Various patterns of endotracheal tubes are available for special requirements, such as thoracic surgery. Endotracheal tubes may be:
   Cuffed or plain
   Designed for oral or nasal use
   Reusable or disposable

Of the various materials used in the manufacture of endotracheal tubes the most common are red rubber and PVC. Red rubber tubes may be sterilized and reused. They are only suitable for relatively short periods of intubation since they cause mucosal irritation. It is sometimes considered false economy to sterilize and reuse tubes, and the cuff will eventually weaken, with the risk that it may fail to inflate when the tube is in position.

Tubes for single use are often made of PVC and are used if the patient is to be intubated for a longer period of time. A PVC tube, often known as a 'Portex' tube, is often used with a Portex connector, made of blue plastic, and a Portex catheter mount.

Tubes for adult use come in a wide range of sizes. Sizes describe the inner diameter of the tube in millimetres. The standard size for a woman of average build would be 8.0 mm or 8.5 mm.

*Connectors*
The connector links the endotracheal tube to the catheter mount. Connectors are right-angled or curved and may or may not have a suction port (Fig. 2.7). A connector with such a port has a bung attached to it, and it is particularly useful in obstetrics since it facilitates the use of an introducer (see Chapter 8: *Difficult Intubation*).

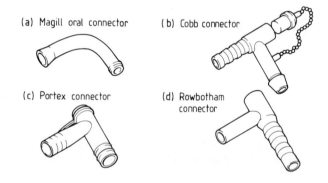

(a) Magill oral connector

(b) Cobb connector

(c) Portex connector

(d) Rowbotham connector

**Fig. 2.7** Endotracheal tube connectors. Various types are available.

*The Catheter Mount*
The catheter mount links the connector to the male end of the anaesthetic or ventilator circuit tubing. It consists of a short, narrow-bore piece

of corrugated tubing with a plain rubber taper at one end. This taper fits onto the connector. At the other end is the standard female fitting.

*Airways*
An airway is used to prevent obstruction of the patient's natural airway whilst she is unconscious. Such obstruction is likely to be caused by the patient's tongue falling back onto the posterior pharyngeal wall, if the patient is supine. The airway may be inserted alongside an endotracheal tube prior to extubation, and it is commonly used during an anaesthetic in which gas is administered via a face mask, with the patient breathing spontaneously.

Two basic types of airway are available. An oral airway is commonly used, though nasal airways are also available. The Guedel airway (Fig. 2.8) is popular. It is made of black rubber or PVC and has a metal insert to prevent occlusion if the patient clenches her teeth during recovery.

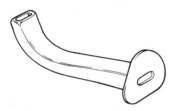

**Fig. 2.8** A Guedel airway.

## OTHER ITEMS OF ANAESTHETIC EQUIPMENT

*Magill's forceps* (Fig. 2.9). These forceps are used in nasal intubation to guide the tip of the endotracheal tube through the vocal cords under direct vision. They may also be used for inserting a throat pack. They are angled in two planes so that the anaesthetist's hand does not obscure his view as he uses them.

*Mouth gags and props.* These are used to keep the patient's mouth open and may occasionally be required. They should be used with care so as not to damage the teeth and should be inserted at the side

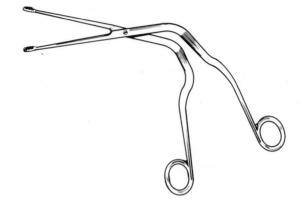

**Fig. 2.9** Magill's forceps.

of the mouth, so that they rest on the molars. The jaws of the unconscious patient must not be forced too widely open.

*Head harness* (Fig. 2.10). Various patterns of harness exist for holding face masks in position on the anaesthetized patient. The anaesthetist will often prefer to hold the mask in position himself since this gives him better opportunity to observe and maintain the patient's airway, but a harness should be available.

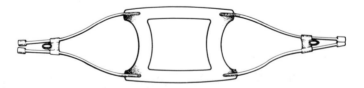

**Fig. 2.10** A head harness, which may be used to hold the mask in position.

*Throat spray.* The Macintosh spray is designed to deliver local anaesthetic solution to the nose prior to nasal intubation, or to the oropharynx and cords for direct laryngoscopy or 'awake intubation' which may occasionally be performed.

Other sundries which should be kept in the anaesthetic room and theatre are syringes, needles, lubricant jelly and gauze swabs. Gauze swabs are usually green to differentiate them from those included in the scrub nurse's swab count. Ideally, they are also X-ray detectable, as are those in the scrub nurse's swab count.

Suction equipment must be available at every point where an unconscious patient may be present. It must be fully equipped and maintained, and must be checked daily.

All necessities for commencing and maintaining an intravenous infusion, including blood transfusion, must be readily available. Monitoring equipment, such as an ECG, and perhaps an automatic blood pressure recorder, will also be needed.

**Ventilators**
Artificial ventilation of the patient will be necessary if she has been given a muscle relaxant. The anaesthetist may ventilate the patient's lungs manually during a short procedure, but more commonly he will use an anaesthetic circuit linked to a ventilator. Gas is delivered under pressure during the inspiratory phase, but the lungs are allowed to empty spontaneously during the expiratory phase. This is termed 'Intermittent Positive Pressure Ventilation' or IPPV.

Ventilators vary in design and appearance, but may be classified as: pressure-cycled, volume-cycled, or time-cycled.

These terms refer to the means used to initiate the action of the bellows. On the inspiratory side of the ventilator circuit, the patient's endotracheal (or tracheostomy) tube is connected to bellows which are filled with the gas to be delivered to the patient. The bellows are emptied by pressure created by a weight, an electric motor, or the gas surrounding them.

The changeover from inspiration to expiration is signalled by:
i) the reaching of a certain pressure within the airways — pressure cycling,
ii) the delivery of a certain (pre-set) volume of gas — volume cycling, or,
iii) the passing of a certain length of time (again pre-set) — time cycling.

Resistance to expiration may be inserted, causing the pressure in the airways to remain above atmospheric pressure instead of falling to atmospheric pressure, which is normal. This is called Positive End Expiratory Pressure (PEEP).

In some of the modern machines a pause is inserted between inspiration and expiration.

Some ventilators, such as the Manley, run solely from the gases being delivered to the patient. Others, such as the Cape, require electricity in addition, and yet others also require a source of compressed air.


## HAZARDS IN THE OPERATING THEATRE

### The Risk of Explosion or Fire
The risk of explosion or fire exists when three factors are present together.
i) The presence of a gas which supports combustion — $O_2$ or $N_2O$, or both.
ii) The presence of flammable substances such as flammable anaesthetic agents or degreasing solution.
iii) A source of ignition.

The prevention of fires and explosions in hospitals has been aimed mainly at removing the third factor. The two main sources of ignition found in operating theatre areas are sparks from electrical apparatus and sparks from an accumulation of static electricity.

*Sparks from electrical apparatus.* Any electrical equipment used within a zone which extends 10 cm around the breathing circuit must be spark-proof. This is not compulsory outside this area, but such equipment should be marked 'NOT TO BE USED WITHIN THE ZONE OF RISK'. This notice replaces the older 'NOT TO BE USED IN THE PRESENCE OF FLAMMABLE ANAESTHETICS'.

*Static electricity.* Sparking from static electricity is prevented by:
i) fairly high relative humidity of the atmosphere in theatre, usually about 67%, and
ii) the use of anti-static materials for breathing circuits, trolley wheels, trolley and table covers, floor covering and footwear. Both staff and patients should wear cotton clothing, and only cotton cellular blankets or sheets are used.

The compression of gases in cylinders generates heat, and this heat may cause an explosion if oil or grease is present on the cylinder valves, particularly in the presence of $O_2$ or $N_2O$.

Although pollution of the theatre atmosphere should be markedly reduced by the use of modern equipment, it is still considered correct to place electrical sockets well above floor level to minimize the risk of sparking which might cause a fire in the presence of an accumulation of flammable gases heavier than air.

Smoking and the use of any naked flame should clearly be strictly prohibited anywhere within the vicinity of the operating area, or, indeed, wherever medical gases are stored.

All staff must be conversant with fire procedures and be aware of the location and use of fire extinguishers.

### Pollution of the Atmosphere

Considerable research has been carried out on the effects of anaesthetic gas pollution on theatre staff, particularly females. It was thought that such pollution may have contributed to a higher incidence of spontaneous abortion in theatre staff who become pregnant, but current thinking does not relate this phenomenon to the inhalation of traces of anaesthetic gases, though the phenomenon does exist.

The DHSS recommends the use of anti-pollution systems which remove all expired gases from the theatre environment to an outlet outside the hospital. Such anti-pollution systems may be active, incorporating an extractor fan, or passive, consisting only of conduits to an outlet.

Most operating theatres today also have air conditioning systems giving several complete air changes in one hour, so that pollution of the atmosphere should be minimized.

### Other Hazards to Theatre Staff

These include radiation and infection, neither of which will be significant in obstetrics. However, serum hepatitis is an important hazard and staff must be familiar with local procedure when a patient who is 'Australia-Antigen positive' is to undergo any operative treatment. All protective measures must be conscientiously applied in this instance. Special consideration is given to hazards to the patient in operating theatres in Chapter 7.

### THE OPERATING TABLE

The operating table is designed to provide a full range of positions so that both anaesthetist and surgeon have easy access to the patient as required. The basic table has a full range of fittings to allow positioning

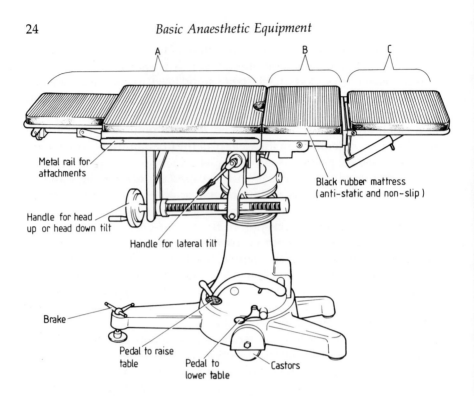

A B C

Metal rail for
attachments

Handle for head
up or head down tilt

Handle for lateral tilt

Black rubber mattress
(anti-static and non-slip)

Brake

Pedal to raise
table

Pedal to
lower table

Castors

**Fig. 2.11** An operating table of the type used in obstetrics and gynaecology. In this model, section C folds down, and section A then slides down over section B towards the operator when the lithotomy position is used.

of the patient (Fig. 2.11), and various special tables are available for specialties such as orthopaedics and neurosurgery.

The theatre table usually consists of a metal base arranged in several sections (often four). The mattress is covered in anti-static rubber, usually ridged or otherwise rendered 'non-slip', so that the patient will not slide if a tilt in any direction is required. The mattress may be removed in sections for cleaning. The table can be raised or lowered, usually by means of a foot pedal. It may tilt to a head-up or head-down position, and the section at either end may also be tilted in either direction. A lateral tilt may also be effected, and the two adjoining central sections may often be 'cracked', i.e. tilted away from each other, for positions such as the 'kidney position'.

Because of its structure, the table is heavy, but is usually fairly easy to manoeuvre on castors. The brake should be on before the table is used. The table must be regularly serviced and maintained.

Fittings for the various attachments and accessories usually slide onto a rail along the edge of the metal base of the table. Such attachments will include arm-boards and lithotomy poles. The anaesthetic screen is a right-angled piece of tubular metal over which the towels may be draped in order to give the anaesthetist access to the patient's face and chest, or to prevent the conscious patient with a regional block from watching the operative procedure. Various supports may be used to keep the patient secure in specialized positions such as the 'kidney position'. Foam pads or pillows, sandbags, or straps may also be used to maintain the patient's position or to prevent pressure on vulnerable nerves or contact with metal (see Chapter 7: *Positioning of the Patient*). Pads and pillows are usually covered with anti-static rubber.

A table for obstetrics is used either in the normal position for abdominal surgery, but with lateral tilt or a buttock wedge for the pregnant patient, or in the lithotomy position. The lithotomy poles may be attached at each side of the table, and care must be taken to ensure that they are symmetrical in angle and height. The bottom sections of the table may be detachable, or they may fold down or slide away under the upper sections.

## SUGGESTED FURTHER READING

Carrie, L. E. S. and Simpson, P. J. (1982) *Understanding Anaesthesia*, 1st edn. London: William Heinemann Medical Books.

Dixon, E. (1983) *Theatre Technique* (Nurses' Aids Series), 5th edn. London: Baillière Tindall.

Grant W. J. (1978) *Medical Gases — Their Properties and Uses*, 1st edn. London: HM&M Publishers.

Wachstein, J. and Smith J. A. H. (1981) *Anaesthesia and Recovery Room Techniques* (Nurses' Aids Series), 3rd edn. London: Baillière Tindall.

Wallace, C. J. (1981) *Anaesthetic Nursing*, 1st edn. London: Pitman Medical.

Ward, C. S. (1975) *Anaesthetic Equipment — Physical Principles and Maintenance*, 1st edn. London: Baillière Tindall.

# 3 Drugs Used in Anaesthesia

## SOME BASIC PRINCIPLES AND DEFINITIONS

Because the needs of the surgical patient and, indeed, of his surgeon are so diverse, the anaesthetist is required to provide the following in varying proportions:

    sleep or hypnosis
    analgesia
    muscle relaxation

These factors are known as the triad of general anaesthesia. Hypnosis and analgesia are implied in the term 'general anaesthesia'. Some degree of muscle relaxation will always be present, but, for example, when endotracheal intubation is required, or in the case of abdominal surgery, more profound relaxation will be necessary.

In the early days, anaesthesia was induced with one of the gaseous or volatile agents. Several stages were then clearly seen. The problem was that, to obtain muscle relaxation, deep anaesthesia had to be given, with attendant respiratory and cardiovascular depression and a prolonged recovery period. Modern techniques mask these stages and enable the anaesthetist to bring the patient quickly and easily through them. Guedel's classic description of the stages of anaesthesia is still of interest and helps in understanding the principles of anaesthesia. The stages of anaesthesia are:

i) **Analgesia.** At induction of anaesthesia the patient becomes unconscious. All reflexes are present, and the patient continues to breathe spontaneously and quietly, though respirations may be irregular.

ii) **Excitement or delirium.** The patient becomes restless, unco-operative and may be violent, though remaining asleep. He or she may retch or vomit. All reflexes are still present.

iii) **Surgical anaesthesia.** The restless stage has passed, and the patient is asleep and breathing quietly. If anaesthesia is allowed to deepen further, the patient passes through the following phases or planes:

*Plane 1:* Respirations are still regular and automatic. The eyelash reflex has gone, and rapid eye movements may be seen.

*Plane 2:* The eyes are fixed. Laryngeal reflexes are no longer present, though the respiratory muscles are still functional.

*Plane 3:* The intercostal muscles are paralysed, and respiration becomes diaphragmatic only. Profound muscle relaxation is seen.

*Plane 4:* Respirations are completely depressed and complete muscle relaxation is seen.

iv) **Medullary paralysis.** The pupils are dilated, the skin cold and pale. The blood pressure falls, the pulse is feeble, and death is imminent and inevitable.

With intravenous induction agents, the patient passes quickly from Stage I to a state of surgical anaesthesia, and this is further facilitated by the use of premedication. However, this would be short-lived if anaesthesia were not maintained. This is usually achieved by using the gaseous agents, for example, nitrous oxide and oxygen with either a volatile or an intravenous supplement. If adequate analgesia is given, and if abolition of reflexes and muscle relaxation is not required, the patient may be kept at this level, breathing spontaneously. If muscle relaxation is required, then it is at this stage that a muscle relaxant is given, endotracheal intubation is performed, and the patient is artificially ventilated. Once the patient is paralysed, anaesthesia must be maintained so that he or she remains asleep and pain-free. If anaesthesia were allowed to become too light, the patient could return to consciousness, be able to hear and feel, but unable to move or indicate his plight because of the action of the muscle relaxant. At a slightly deeper level, the patient may be asleep, but may respond to painful stimuli such as traction on the peritoneum. Such response is seen as an increase in heart rate, raised blood pressure or even a slight movement. There is no recall of such response, but as well as hypnosis, the patient does require adequate analgesia.

Clearly the anaesthetist is required to keep the patient in optimum condition, and adequate oxygenation and hydration are essential. Avoidance, as far as possible, of iatrogenic morbidity or drug interaction is also an important consideration, particularly when the patient is receiving any other drug therapy.

Revision of basic terminology may be helpful at this point.

**Analgesia** — absence of pain.

**Anaesthesia** — absence of feeling. General anaesthesia implies total absence of feeling, in other words, loss of consciousness, and freedom from pain. It is a drug-induced, reversible state. Regional anaesthetic techniques may give a combination of analgesia and anaesthesia. Thus epidural analgesia may give a small area of anaesthesia, where all sensation is lost, with a greater area which is pain-free, but where sensations of touch, although altered, are still present. It is important that the patient understands this before surgery under regional block is performed.

**'Crash Induction'** — a method of inducing general anaesthesia whereby the risk of inhalation of regurgitated stomach contents is minimized. Ideally, the surgical patient should be starved for at least four hours pre-operatively, but the patient's condition may be such that immediate surgery is essential. Stress may delay gastric emptying, and the patient may be unable to provide information as to when he last ate or drank. When stomach contents may be present, so that there is a danger of vomiting or regurgitation during induction of anaesthesia, with aspiration of acid material into the lungs, 'crash induction' is performed. The airway is protected from stomach contents by the use of cricoid pressure and endotracheal intubation. This is discussed in detail in Chapters 4 and 7.

**Neuroleptanaesthesia** — a dissociative anaesthetic technique in which the patient is given sedation, is pain free and detached from reality without losing vital reflexes or becoming uncontrollable.

**Narcotic Drugs** — the word 'narcotic' is derived from the Greek word meaning 'stupor', and refers to drugs that produce insensibility. Commonly, this means drugs that induce sleep and which may also induce analgesia, and usually refers either to the opiates, which induce both, or to the barbiturates which induce sleep only. The former will therefore give two of the components of the anaesthetic triad, and indeed large doses of an opiate, together with a muscle relaxant, may be used to induce anaesthesia for cardiac surgery. It is important to differentiate between the legal and pharmacological use of the word 'narcotic', in order to avoid confusion. The former refers to drugs of addiction, such as cocaine, LSD and marijuana, as well as morphine and heroin.

**Sedatives** — a sedative is a drug which induces calmness, and this will often lead to sleep.

**Hypnotic Drugs** — an hypnotic drug produces drowsiness and will facilitate the onset and maintenance of a state resembling natural sleep, from which the recipient may be easily aroused.

**Tranquillizers** — these are drugs which relieve anxiety and which in larger doses will often induce sleep.

The differences between sedatives, hypnotics and tranquillizers are often not clearly defined. Sedatives, hypnotics and general anaesthetics generally produce increasing depths of depression of the central nervous system, and, in fact, sedatives and hypnotics in large doses do produce general anaesthesia. It is important to remember that hypnotics have no analgesic effect, and will not induce sleep in the presence of severe pain. In this situation, disorientation and loss of self-control often occurs.

A selection of drugs commonly used in general anaesthesia will now be considered.

## PREMEDICATION

The aim of premedication of the surgical patient is generally two-fold.

### Anxiolysis
A relaxed, often sleepy patient will experience less stress, and induction of anaesthesia is usually quicker and easier. Sedative premedication will prolong post-operative drowsiness, and is not always desirable, for example, in day-case surgery.

### Vagal blockade
Stimulation of the vagus may cause a situation known as vagal inhibition, in which there may be extreme bradycardia. When associated with, for example, hypoxia, cardiac arrest may occur. Such stimulation may occur in ophthalmic surgery, anal dilatation or endotracheal intubation. The use of atropine in premedication helps to prevent undesirable vagal reflexes. The vagal blocking drugs which dry up secretions are known as antisialogogues, and those in common use are atropine, hyoscine (Scopolamine) and glycopyrrolate (Robinul). Drying of secretions, both salivary and bronchial, is helpful for the anaesthetist, though sometimes unpleasant for the patient.

## INDUCTION AGENTS

Various drugs are used intravenously to induce anaesthesia. They have a rapid onset of action, and the aim in using them is to cause easy transition into unconsciousness in a few seconds. They are metabolized and either excreted or redistributed within the body over a short period of time, so that within minutes the patient will regain consciousness unless anaesthesia is maintained by giving the intravenous agent in titrated doses or by continuous intravenous infusion, or most commonly, by using the inhalational anaesthetic agents.

## Thiopentone (Pentothal, Intraval)

First introduced in 1934, this is probably still the most widely used induction agent. In doses of 4.5 mg/kg, it produces smooth induction in about 20 seconds, and its action, which lasts about 5–10 minutes, is terminated by its redistribution within body tissues, though excretion is not completed for several hours. It is slowly metabolized by the liver, giving a 'hangover' effect. Thiopentone may cause respiratory depression and hypotension. Asthmatic patients may develop broncho-spasm, and laryngospasm may occur if the larynx is stimulated by the presence of sputum, vomitus, blood or an airway. Inadvertent intra-arterial injection may cause distal necrosis, and extra-vascular injection may cause considerable localized irritation and even tissue necrosis. The occurrence of either event will cause pain on injection. It should not be given to patients with a history of barbiturate sensitivity or to patients who suffer from porphyria.

## Methohexitone (Brietal)

This again is a barbiturate similar to thiopentone with rapid onset and short duration of action. It gives pleasant, easy induction, though the patient may complain of pain in the arm as it is injected. Immediately after induction the patient may cough, hiccup, or become hypertonic. These are known as the excitatory phenomena. They may be severe enough to cause convulsions, and methohexitone is not usually given to patients with any predisposition to convulsions.

## Althesin (Alphaloxone)

This is not a barbiturate, but a mixture of steroid drugs, though without any steroid effects. It has an oily base — Cremophor E, and is difficult to inject quickly. Generally speaking, it causes litle respiratory or cardio-vascular depression, but may, quite unpredictably, cause dramatic hypersensitivity. Althesin is one of the drugs more commonly used to maintain anaesthesia for short procedures, as well as for induction.

### Ketamine (Ketalar)

This drug may be used in dissociative techniques where reflexes are not necessarily abolished, but good sedation and analgesia are achieved. It may cause hypertension and tachycardia. Its main disadvantage is that it may be hallucinogenic, though the incidence of this is said to be reduced following premedication. The nightmares may be extremely distressing, and patients who have received ketamine should be allowed to recover in a quiet room. It does not appear to produce this problem in small children.

### Propanidid (Epontol)

This is a non-barbiturate agent with the same base as Althesin. On injection, it may cause hyperventilation followed by apnoea, and it causes more marked cardiovascular depression than the other induction agents. It has a very short duration of action. It is associated with a significant incidence of allergic reactions.

### Etomidate (Hypnomidate)

This is another non-barbiturate induction agent. It causes little cardiovascular depression, but injection may be painful, and there is a high incidence of excitatory phenomena.

## MAINTENANCE AGENTS

### The Anaesthetic Gases

### Nitrous Oxide (N₂O)

This is a sweet-smelling, colourless gas. It is not flammable but does support combustion if the temperature is high enough to decompose it into nitrogen and oxygen. It is a good analgesic, but not a potent anaesthetic agent, and is used together with a volatile or an intravenous supplement. Nitrous oxide is relatively non-toxic, having little adverse effect on the respiratory or cardiovascular systems. If breathed for 24 hours or more, it can be associated with changes in the bone marrow. If breathed for shorter periods, as in intensive care, it is associated with changes in the red cells, from interference with vitamin $B_{12}$.

## Oxygen ($O_2$)

Ordinary air contains 20.9% of oxygen, and adequate oxygenation is a vital part of any anaesthetic procedure. It is given at rates higher than 21%, however, because with changes in the lungs occurring during anaesthesia, the oxygen tension in the blood would fall if oxygen were given at this rate. For this reason, it is usual to increase the flow of oxygen to 30–33% of the breathing mixture.

## Carbon Dioxide ($CO_2$)

This colourless gas is found in air in a concentration of 0.03%. It is a product of metabolism in the body, and normal ventilation is required to remove it. Where respiration is depressed, the $CO_2$ level in the blood rises, and this can be associated with serious side-effects, such as cardiac arrhythmias. For a time, it was thought appropriate to keep $CO_2$ at a low level in the blood, and this was part of anaesthetic practice. Normocarbia — $CO_2$ at a tension of 40 mm of mercury in the blood — is now thought to be the ideal. Carbon dioxide is occasionally used during an anaesthetic to stimulate the respiratory centre and deepen respiration in order to increase uptake of gaseous agents in a gaseous induction and so speed up the process, or to deepen respiration as an aid to 'blind' intubation, usually nasal. At the end of an anaesthetic, it may be given to stimulate the respiratory centre when the patient has been mechanically ventilated, with a resulting fall in $PCO_2$.

## Cyclopropane ($C_3H_6$)

Cyclopropane is not commonly used in the UK today. Its main disadvantages are its expense and its flammability. Because it is expensive, it is used in a closed circuit, where much reduced fresh gas flow is required. It may not be used with diathermy because of its flammability. It is, however, a potent anaesthetic agent. Low concentrations are used, so that the patient may also receive higher concentrations of oxygen. It gives rapid induction of anaesthesia, and so may be useful in paediatric anaesthesia. It gives a significant incidence of cardiac arrhythmias and also of post-operative nausea and vomiting.

## The Volatile Agents

The volatile agents may be used with oxygen as induction agents, particularly for children.

*Halothane (Fluothane)*
This is frequently used as a supplement to nitrous oxide and oxygen. It gives good hypnosis and relaxation, but not analgesia. It gives rapid induction and recovery. However, it does depress the myocardium, and reduces peripheral resistance, so that hypotension may occur. Brady- cardia may also be seen when it is used. Although widely used in general surgery, it is generally inappropriate for use in obstetric anaesthe- sia in anything other than low concentrations, since it causes relaxation of the myometrium and will therefore tend to cause increased blood loss at caesarean section. A feature of recovery from halothane may be 'halothane shakes', which has no clinical significance and resolves spontaneously, though it may be reversed by giving an intravenous analgesic or by giving methyl-phenidate. Halothane is very occasionally related to post-operative hepatitis, particularly after repeated administ- ration in subsequent anaesthetics, though the exact aetiology is not clear.

*Trichloroethylene (Trilene)*
This is discussed in Chapter 11 as an inhalational analgesic agent. In nitrous oxide and oxygen as its carrier gas it gives good analgesia, but relatively poor hypnosis. It may cause cardiac arrhythmias and hypo- tension. It is not used in a closed circuit with soda lime, since the two may produce toxic substances.

*Enflurane (Ethrane)*
This relatively new agent is similar in many ways to halothane. Again, it is not a good analgesic, though it gives good hypnosis and relaxation. It does not affect liver function in the same way as halothane is thought to do; it is not metabolized to the same extent but is excreted almost unchanged. This is seen as its main advantage. It has a depressant effect on both respiratory and cardiovascular systems.

*Methoxyflurane (Penthrane)*
This agent was in use for a while; it is more potent than the other volatile agents, but was not easy to use as an anaesthetic supplement, since it does not readily vaporize. It has prolonged induction and recovery times, and is associated with renal toxicity, producing high levels of fluoride ions which are formed during its metabolism. It is no longer approved for anaesthetic use in the UK, but is an effective inhalational

analgesic for obstetrics and painful procedures such as burns dressings, which have to be performed repeatedly.

## Ether
Unlike the other volatile agents, ether gives all three components of anaesthesia — hypnosis, analgesia and relaxation. However, both induction and recovery are prolonged, and it gives a high incidence of nausea and vomiting. It is also explosive. It was very popular in the past, because it gave sufficient relaxation for abdominal surgery without such deep anaesthesia that respiratory depression and arrest would occur. Furthermore, respiratory depression occurred before cardiovascular depression, making it relatively safe. In obstetrics it was popular because it gave analgesia and relaxation at a level where laryngeal reflexes were still present, making it relatively safe if regurgitation occurred. It is cheap to manufacture and is used in the underdeveloped countries.

## Chloroform
Chloroform was popular as an induction agent in the early days of anaesthesia, as the onset of anaesthesia was more rapid than with ether. Two properties in particular were responsible for its withdrawal from modern anaesthesia. It tends to cause severe cardiac arrhythmias, particularly ventricular fibrillation, probably because it sensitizes the heart to the effects of adrenaline, levels of which would be high in apprehensive individuals. It is also toxic to the liver, the toxicity being due to a breakdown product of the vapour.

## MUSCLE RELAXANTS

Muscle relaxants are described according to their mode of action at the neuromuscular junction. An understanding of the mechanism of neuromuscular transmission is essential here. The transmission of nervous impulses is a form of electrical activity. At the point where the nerve fibre meets the muscle is a minute gap known as the synaptic cleft or gutter. The muscle fibres form the 'motor end plate', and the nervous impulse must cross the synapse in order to activate the muscle. A stimulus reaching the nerve ending causes release of acetylcholine, which diffuses across the synapse and attaches itself to the receptor cells on the motor end plate. The release of acetylcholine causes a change in the ratio of sodium and potassium ions across the motor end plate. This electrical activity is called depolarization and causes the muscle to contract. As this occurs, the acetylcholine is broken down by an enzyme called acetylcholinesterase. The muscle fibre then enters a brief refractory or resting phase, after which the process may recur. This whole process occurs over perhaps 1/500 of a second.

The two types of muscle relaxant are known as the depolarizing and non-depolarizing relaxants. The former act by maintaining a state of depolarization. They are similar to acetylcholine, but are broken down by pseudocholinesterase, and as this is a much more prolonged action than that occurring in the motor end plate, the state of paralysis persists for minutes rather than only a fraction of a second. The non-depolarizing agents act by competing for the acetylcholine receptor cells on the motor end plate, thus preventing diffusion of acetylcholine across the synapse. They are sometimes therefore known as the 'competitive relaxants'.

### Depolarizing Relaxants

The 'depolarizer' in current use is suxamethonium (Scoline). Its onset of action is rapid, occurring within seconds, and its effect lasts for about 3–5 minutes. There is no known antidote at present, and prolonged action — 'Scoline apnoea' — occurs very occasionally. This problem arises if there is a deficiency or some abnormality of the patient's pseudo-cholinesterase. Such phenomena may be familial, and it is usual to investigate relatives if the problem occurs. Suxamethonium is given prior to intubation, since complete relaxation occurs within seconds. Fasciculation (generalized twitching of the muscles) precedes relaxation. The administration of suxamethonium may cause generalized muscle pains post-operatively, and the patient may require mild analgesia for these. Suxamethonium is sometimes given in incremental doses — 'inter-mittent suxamethonium' — or by means of a continuous intravenous infusion.

### Non-depolarizing Relaxants

These are effective within 3–4 minutes, and give relaxation for periods of 20–40 minutes. They are given following intubation, so that their action continues when that of suxamethonium has worn off. They may be given as necessary, often in reduced doses, and once their effect has begun to tail off, they may be reversed.

*D-Tubocurarine (Tubarine).* A pure preparation of curare. It may cause hypotension, or in susceptible patients, bronchospasm. It gives relaxation for about 30–40 minutes.

*Pancuronium (Pavulon)*. A steroid-type drug with minimal side effects. It is often used for the patient who is being artificially ventilated for other than anaesthetic reasons. Its onset of action is rapid, and relaxation is maintained for 25–35 minutes.

*Alcuronium (Alloferin)*. A synthetic agent with similar properties to pancuronium.

*Gallamine (Flaxedil)*. This was one of the first synthetic relaxants. It tends to produce a tachycardia. Because of its slightly stimulant effect on the cardiovascular system, blood pressure is well maintained. It crosses the placental barrier to a greater extent than the other relaxant agents.

*Fazadinium (Fazadon)*. This drug has been produced fairly recently, its advantage being rapid onset and shorter duration of action, but it has not in fact replaced the other non-depolarizers to any great extent.

*Atracurium (Tracrium)*. A newly introduced drug of medium duration of action, having little, if any, adverse effect on the cardiovascular system. It does not depend on the liver or kidney for its elimination, and is therefore likely to be very useful in patients with diminished renal function.

## Reversal Agents
The action of non-depolarizing relaxants may be reversed, provided a repeat dose has not just been given. If the non-depolarizer competes with the acetylcholine receptors, so denying access to acetylcholine, its reversal is effected by increasing production of acetylcholine, so that in turn it may compete for its own receptors. This increased production of acetylcholine occurs when secretion of acetylcholinesterase is blocked, thus preventing the breakdown of acetylcholine. The drug used to inhibit production of acetylcholinesterase is neostigmine (Prostigmine). Neostigmine stimulates the parasympathetic nervous system, causing excessive salivation, bradycardia and increased gut activity. Atropine produces parasympathetic blockade and so counteracts these undesirable side-effects. For this reason neostigmine and atropine are used together to reverse the non-depolarizers. One potential problem is that the effect of neostigmine may wear off before the muscle relaxant has been completely excreted, when 'recurarization' may occur. Neostigmine is one

of the anticholinesterase group of drugs, and others include pyridostigmine, physostigmine and edrophonium (Tensilon).

## NARCOTICS AND ANALGESICS

These drugs are used before, during and after anaesthesia, to produce analgesia, sedation and euphoria. The opiates are probably the most used group despite the problems of respiratory depression and nausea. There are various synthetic opiates which have been developed in recent years, which may be given in larger doses with relatively less severe side-effects; in other words their therapeutic ratio is wider. These include fentanyl (Sublimaze) and phenoperidine (Operidine). An intravenous opiate is often used as a supplement to general anaesthesia, and the advantage of this is that a degree of analgesia will continue to be present in the immediate post-operative period.

### Morphine
This is the standard strong analgesic, which still retains its use in medicine despite its side-effects. It has useful euphoric properties, and although addiction is a possibility, this should not be a problem when the drug is given for the relief of pain associated with surgery. It is a respiratory depressant, and causes nausea and vomiting and also constriction of plain muscle in the gut, bronchi and other organs. It releases histamine, and this, with its bronchoconstrictor properties, makes it unsuitable for use in asthmatics. Hypotension may occur. Its duration of action is 3–4 hours, following a standard intramuscular dose of 10–15 mg.

### Diamorphine (Heroin)
Twice as potent, but with similar effects to morphine, diamorphine gives excellent analgesia. Its potency is explained by the fact that it is converted to morphine in the body. Dosage is 5–7 mg intramuscularly.

### Pethidine
This is a synthetic opiate similar to morphine, differing in that it causes relaxation of smooth muscle rather than constriction. It is therefore useful for patients with renal or biliary colic, and for asthmatics. It produces less euphoria and sedation, and has a shorter duration of action. Dosage is 50–150 mg intramuscularly.

## Papaveretum (Omnopon)

This is a mixture of opium alkaloids, containing 50% dried morphine and about 50% codeine. 15 mg is equivalent to 10 mg morphine sulphate. Its action and side effects are similar to those of morphine.

## Fentanyl (Sublimaze)

A synthetic opiate similar to pethidine, fentanyl is popular as an intra-operative analgesic. Its duration of action is dependent on the dose given, and dosage varies considerably — from 3 to 100 $\mu$g/kg. Fentanyl is a potent respiratory depressant but has few other side-effects. The heart rate tends to fall, following an intravenous dose, but the blood pressure remains steady, even after larger doses.

## Phenoperidine (Operidine)

Another synthetic analgesic related to pethidine, phenoperidine has a longer duration of action than fentanyl. It tends to cause hypotension. It is often used to provide sedation and respiratory depression in patients receiving artificial ventilation in intensive therapy units.

## Opiate Antagonists

The majority of drugs produce their effect by combining with specialized areas of cell membrane known as receptors. The opiate drugs, for example, act by combining with opiate receptors found on the cell membranes of many nerve cells, including those associated with the transmission of pain, but also those responsible for initiating nausea and vomiting and those associated with the control of respiration. Opiate receptors are also found in the gut, explaining the action of these drugs on this organ.

An agonist drug is one that combines with its receptors, causing a pharmacological effect.

An antagonist drug is one that also combines with specific receptors, often more easily than an agonist drug, but this combination is followed by diminished or no effect.

A drug giving diminished effect is known as a mixed agonist/antagonist drug.

Until recently, the available opiate antagonist drugs also had agonist properties, and, if given without an opiate, would produce morphine-like effects. Antagonism was only produced if the antagonist was given to a patient who had already received an opiate. Nalorphine (Lethidrone) and levallorphan (Lorfan) are examples. Although these drugs reversed the respiratory depressant effects of opiates, they also reduced the analgesia.

More recently, naloxone (Narcan) has been introduced. This is a pure antagonist if given on its own. Given in the absence of an opiate, it has no morphine-like effects, in other words, it has no agonist action. It antagonizes both the respiratory depressant and analgesic effect of the opiates, but has a relatively short duration of action, so there is always a danger of 'renarcotization' when its action ceases.

### Mixed Agonist/Antagonist Analgesics

The search for a potent analgesic without addictive or respiratory depressant properties has been largely unsuccessful so far. Drugs in this category have been unsatisfactory for other reasons. Some, for example, have caused hallucinations or disorientation. An example of this type of drug is pentazocine (Fortral).

### Other Analgesics

The drugs already discussed act directly on the central nervous system, blocking nerve impulses along the pain pathways running between the spinal cord and the thalamus. They also affect the emotional response to pain. Other, milder analgesics, such as aspirin and paracetamol, act peripherally by an action thought to involve inhibition of prostaglandins. These substances are synthesized throughout the body and are produced locally as required, have an effect and are rapidly destroyed. Prostaglandins are thought to be involved in the process occurring between a painful stimulus and the initiation of an impulse in a nerve fibre relaying pain. A mixture of an opiate and a mild analgesic, such as morphine and aspirin, is more effective than either drug used alone.

## LOCAL ANAESTHETIC AGENTS

Local anaesthetic drugs will be considered at this point, since regional techniques are often performed in conjunction with general anaesthesia in order to provide effective post-operative analgesia and to reduce analgesic requirements during general anaesthesia.

They are used extensively in obstetrics, both by midwives and obstetricians performing local infiltration of the perineum for episiotomy and suturing, and by medical staff performing pudendal blocks and epidural and spinal blocks. An understanding of the pharmacology of local anaesthetic drugs is essential to their safe use; it is also very interesting. The mode of action of local anaesthetic agents relates to depolarization, which was briefly described earlier in this chapter.

Local anaesthesia is a reversible blockade of nervous impulses along nerve fibres. In its resting state the outside of the nerve cell membrane is positively charged relative to the inside, but when a nerve impulse travels along the fibre, the outside transiently becomes negative and the inside positive — depolarization. This is due to a sudden increase in the permeability of the cell membrane to sodium, which rushes into the cell through special channels, carrying its positive charge with it. The entry of sodium displaces potassium, which diffuses out through the cell membrane. The normal equilibrium of sodium and potassium ions is restored by the action of the sodium pump which returns sodium to the extracellular fluid. This restores the resting state of the nerve cell. The process of depolarization occurs repeatedly along the length of the nerve fibre, and at the neuromuscular junction it activates a neurotransmitter; acetylcholine is the example already described, and its release causes contraction of the muscle.

Many different substances will produce local anaesthesia if applied close to nerve fibres. Some of the anti-histamine drugs, the cardiovascular drug propranolol, and pethidine, all have local anaesthetic properties. The application of cold (cryoanalgesia), and pressure on a nerve trunk have similar effects. The local anaesthetic drugs currently in clinical use act by blocking the action of the sodium pump during depolarization. They penetrate the cell membrane and block the sodium channels. Most of these drugs have names ending with the suffix '-aine'. There are two main groups of such drugs, the ester and the amide group:

*The ester group*
  Procaine (Novocain)
  Dibucaine (Nupercaine)
  Tetracaine (Amethocaine)
  Chloroprocaine
*The amide group*
  Lignocaine (Xylocaine)
  Mepivacaine (Carboocaine)
  Prilocaine (Citanest)
  Bupivacaine (Marcain)
  Etidocaine

The basic difference between the two groups is related to their metabolism and their allergic potential. Ester agents are broken down in the plasma by pseudocholinesterase, the enzyme which also breaks down suxamethonium. The amide drugs are metabolized in the liver. One of the principal metabolites of the ester group of drugs is para-aminobenzoic acid (PABA), which is responsible for the occasional allergic type reaction. Amides are not broken down to PABA, and rarely produce an allergic reaction. Many of the so-called allergic reactions to local anaesthetic drugs are in fact due to the absorption of adrenaline which is often added to these drugs, or to preservatives in the solution. The potency of a local anaesthetic agent is related to its solubility in fat. Its duration of action is related to its degree of protein binding; the greater its protein binding the longer its duration of action.

Solutions of commercially available local anaesthetic agents are relatively acid, with a pH of less than 7.00, but to be effective, they need to be made more alkaline. This occurs following injection into the tissues. The more alkaline or basic form of the drug penetrates the nerve cell membrane more easily, and so blocks the sodium channels more effectively. Injection of local anaesthetic drugs into infected or inflamed tissue is ineffective because inflamed tissue is more acid than normal tissue.

The majority of local anaesthetics cause vasodilation, with the exception of cocaine, which causes vasoconstriction, and lignocaine, which causes neither vasoconstriction nor vasodilation. This vasodilator action increases absorption of the drug into the bloodstream, thereby reducing the amount available to act on the nerves. For this reason a vasoconstrictor such as adrenaline or phenylephrine may be added to the local anaesthetic, so as to increase the effectiveness of the block and reduce toxicity. Usually, though not always, the addition of adrenaline results in a more profound and longer lasting block.

The toxicity of local anaesthetic agents depends on the amount passing into the circulation. The following factors affect this:

i) *Dosage.* Obviously the larger the dose, the more drug is likely to be absorbed. The important factor is total dose rather than volume or concentration. 100 mg lignocaine is equally potentially toxic whether given as 10 ml of a 1% solution or 20 ml of 0.5% solution.

ii) *Site of injection.* Local anaesthetics are absorbed more rapidly from some sites than from others. Using the same dose of a local anaesthetic drug, intercostal block gives the highest and subcutaneous injection the lowest blood level, with lumbar epidural block somewhere in between.

iii) *The addition of a vasoconstrictor.* The addition of adrenaline 1: 200 000 significantly reduces blood levels of several agents following peripheral nerve block, but has little effect following lumbar epidural block.

iv) *The agent used.* The rate and degree of absorption varies from one agent to another, causing variations in potency.

The toxic effects of local anaesthetic agents primarily involve the central nervous and cardiovascular systems. The first sign of toxicity is often numbness of the tongue and around the mouth, followed by complaints of a feeling of light-headedness, dizziness and tinnitus. Slurring of speech, drowsiness and muscle twitching may then occur and may progress to generalized convulsions. This is followed by unconsciousness, cardiovascular collapse and respiratory arrest. Treatment consists of support of the cardiovascular and respiratory systems, together with anti-convulsant therapy (often diazepam). Lignocaine and procaine often do not produce the premonitory signs of toxicity, and the first sign is often drowsiness.

The cardiovascular effects of local anaesthetics result either from a direct effect of the drug, or are secondary to a blockade of the sympathetic nervous system. The mode of action inhibiting depolarization can also affect cardiac muscle fibres. At less than toxic doses, lignocaine in particular is effective in preventing abnormal ventricular action, especially ventricular extrasystoles. At toxic doses, however, it will depress the myocardium, causing a fall in cardiac output and blood pressure.

Hypotension may also be a result of sympathetic blockade, particularly following epidural and spinal blocks (see Chapters 12 and 13).

Not all nerve fibres are equally sensitive to local anaesthetics. As a general rule, thinner fibres are more sensitive than thicker ones. This means that a differential block may be produced by using a low concentration of a local anaesthetic agent, which will penetrate the thinner fibres, leaving the thicker fibres relatively unaffected. Pain and temperature sensation are transmitted by thinner nerve fibres, while touch and pressure are carried by thick fibres. Thus analgesia may be produced without total anaesthesia. Motor nerves are among the thickest, so a sensory block with little or no weakness or paralysis may be produced using low concentrations of local anaesthetics. Where muscle relaxation for abdominal surgery is required, high concentrations will be used. Some local anaesthetic agents in common use are:

## Cocaine

The only naturally occurring local anaesthetic still in clinical use, its stimulating effect on the central nervous system produced by the use of low concentrations is responsible for its addictive potential. It is the only local anaesthetic to cause vasoconstriction; this is due to its potentiating effect on catecholamines (adrenaline and noradrenaline). This may lead to severe cardiac arrhythmias. Its main use today is as a topical application, as a spray onto the larynx or as a paste used to anaesthetize the nasal mucosa for surgery on the nose.

## Lignocaine (Xylocaine, Lidocaine)

Lignocaine is effective used topically, infiltrated, or injected epidurally or spinally. Its action is intensified and prolonged by the addition of adrenaline. Maximum safe doses are, 200 mg without adrenaline (20 ml of a 1% solution) and 500 mg with added adrenaline.

## Bupivacaine (Marcain)

This is a popular drug with a long duration of action. It is not effective topically, but is used in plexus blocks and intravenous regional analgesia such as Bier's block. When used for epidural block its action is not so prolonged, and the addition of adrenaline does not affect it in this instance. The recommended maximum safe dose is 2 mg/kg of body weight.

## Cinchocaine (Nupercaine) and Amethocaine (Tetracaine, Pontocaine)

These are used mainly for spinal block. Both are available in dextrose to render them hyperbaric, that is, to give them a specific gravity greater than that of the cerebrospinal fluid. This means that the spread of the solution and the level of the block may be influenced by appropriate positioning of the patient (see also Chapter 13).

The local anaesthetic agent of the future will ideally be required to have a prolonged duration of action, which may be measured in days rather than hours, without any adverse effect on nerve fibres. This would allow post-operative analgesia to be given with one injection of local anaesthetic.

## SUGGESTED FURTHER READING

Atkinson, R. S., Rushman, G. B. and Lee, A. J. (1977) *A Synopsis of Anaesthesia*, 8th edn. Bristol: John Wright.

British Medical Association, Pharmacological Society of Great Britain (1983) *British National Formulary*.

Carrie, L. E. S. and Simpson, P. J. (1982) *Understanding Anaesthesia*, 1st edn. London: Heinemann Medical Books.

Grant, W. J. (1978) *Medical Gases — Their Properties and Uses*, 1st edn. London: HM&M Publishers.

Trounce, J. R. (1981) *Clinical Pharmacology for Nurses*. Edinburgh: Churchill Livingstone.

Vickers, M. D., Wood-Smith, F. G. and Stewart, H. C. (1978) *Drugs in Anaesthetic Practice*. London: Butterworth.

Wallace, C. J. (1981) *Anaesthetic Nursing*, 1st edn. London: Pitman Medical.

Zuck, D. (1969) *The Principles of Anaesthesia for Nurses*. London: Pitman Medical.

# 4 *Obstetric Physiology and Pharmacology*

For nine months the pregnant woman carries a unique type of parasite within her. In order to nourish the growing fetus and remove its waste products as well as to service the growing uterus, various changes occur in the maternal physiology. These changes will now be considered alongside the factors affecting the passage of substances, both natural and pharmacological, across the placenta.

## PHYSIOLOGY IN PREGNANCY

### The Respiratory System
The main changes here are an increase in the size of the thoracic cage, elevation of the diaphragm and an increase in ventilation of about 40%. The first two changes might be thought to be a mechanical effect of upward pressure from the gravid uterus, but in fact they occur before the uterus attains a significant size. The hyperventilation not only serves to increase the uptake of oxygen necessary to supply the fetus, the uterus, and the extra work of the respiratory and cardiovascular systems, but to eliminate carbon dioxide produced by the fetus. Hyperventilation causes a fall in the retention of carbon dioxide in the blood ($PCO_2$), allowing a gradient to develop between fetus and mother. The carbon dioxide moves along the concentration gradient and thereby leaves the fetal circulation.

### Blood Volume
Blood volume rises dramatically during pregnancy. Plasma volume increases by up to 50%, whilst the red cell mass increases less (about 18%), so that there is haemodilution. The increase in plasma volume is greater in multigravidae than in primigravidae, and is also directly related to the number of fetuses. Thus a woman having quads has twice the normal plasma volume. There is a similar relationship with

red cell mass. On the other hand, there is an inverse relationship between haemoglobin level and the size of the baby. A haemoglobin level in the upper range of normal is likely to be associated with a small baby.

### The Cardiovascular System

The cardiac output, usually 5 litres per minute, rises during pregnancy to a peak of 6.5 litres per minute at about 32 weeks; it remains at this level until term. A significant amount of the extra output obviously goes to the enlarging uterus, but there is also increased flow to the skin, gut and kidneys. The heart rate increases by about 15 beats per minute.

In the third trimester, the gravid uterus is of such a size that, with the mother on her back, it obstructs the flow in the abdominal aorta and the inferior vena cava. This leads to decreased venous return and then to reduced  cardiac output. This, in turn, causes impairment of placental blood flow. Aortocaval occlusion or supine hypotensive syndrome may be concealed when compensatory mechanisms are adequate, or revealed if they are not, and maternal blood pressure falls. This problem is further discussed in Chapter 8.

### The Renal System

The kidney receives an increased blood flow during pregnancy. Increased renal function occurs, with an increase in glomerular filtration rate by up to 60%, and a similar increase in tubular reabsorption, so that fluid and electrolyte balances are maintained.

### Changes during Labour

During contractions the cardiac output increases slightly if the patient is in the lateral position. At the height of a contraction there is obstruction of the aorta and common iliac vessels, which is probably responsible for the changes in fetal heart rate which occur. Immediately after delivery there is a further increase in cardiac output, due to increased venous return from the uterus as it contracts. After the third stage there is an immediate drop in requirement within the uterine vessels, and blood is expelled into the general circulation. By one hour following delivery, the cardiovascular changes begin to return to normal, hence the increased urinary output following delivery. The cardiovascular system has returned to normal by about two weeks postpartum.

The acidity of maternal blood increases during the first stage of labour, and becomes more marked during the second stage in mothers given conventional (narcotic and inhalational) analgesia. Those given an epidural block show no acidosis unless they voluntarily push in the second stage. The fetus, however, develops acidosis, the degree of which is related to the length of the second stage. At delivery the degree of acidosis is similar whether the mother received conventional or epidural analgesia. This is because although fetuses of mothers receiving epidural analgesia are less acidotic at the start of the second stage they tend to remain in it longer. There is therefore no justification for the belief that women with an epidural can be left almost indefinitely at full dilatation.

## PLACENTAL TRANSFER

The situation in pregnancy is unique in that the drug given to one individual, the mother, can affect another, the fetus, and this must always be borne in mind by the doctor prescribing drugs. Unfortunately the effect on the fetus is usually of an adverse nature, though not necessarily of clinical importance. The positive aspect of this is that drugs may be given via the mother to treat the fetus. An example would be the use of phenobarbitone to reduce the level of physiological jaundice in the baby, and, more recently, the use of steroids in premature labour to reduce the incidence and severity of respiratory distress syndrome in the infant.

### The Placental Barrier

The tissue separating the mother from the fetus is of course the placenta. In the placenta, maternal and fetal blood come into close approximation, but they are always separated by at least two layers of cells. These layers constitute the placental barrier, across which both vital nutrients for the fetus and its waste products, but also drugs, can pass.

### F/M Ratios

Some idea of how easily a substance will cross the placental barrier can be obtained by simultaneously measuring the level of the substance in the umbilical vein and the maternal blood. The results are expressed as the ratio of fetal blood level to maternal level — the F/M ratio. A ratio of 1.0 indicates equal levels in fetal and maternal blood and therefore no barrier to that particular substance. Levels of less than 1.0 suggest some restriction of passage, and the lower the figure, the greater the barrier.

It is probably true to say that all drugs cross the placenta to some extent. The placental barrier is similar in many respects to the barrier between the blood and the brain, and a good rule of thumb is that all drugs affecting the central nervous system are likely to have the facility of passing from mother to fetus. All analgesics used in labour and all general anaesthetics act on the central nervous system, so that the search for the ideal analgesic in labour seems unlikely to be successful at the present time. However, further developments relating to endogenous opiates may prove to be an important factor in this search in the future.

*Diffusion*

This is simply the name of the process whereby a substance moves from an area where it is present in high concentration to an area where it is present in lower concentration, through a membrane which is permeable to that substance. In other words, it moves along its concentration gradient. A drug administered to the mother causes a certain level of that drug to be present in the maternal blood. As there is initially none of that drug in the fetal blood it crosses the placenta along its concentration gradient. This process continues until the level of the drug is the same on both sides of the placenta. If the level of the drug in the fetal blood rises above that in the maternal blood, diffusion will occur in the opposite direction, as with carbon dioxide, for example. Intravenous administration of a drug to the mother leads to a rapid rise in maternal blood concentration, favouring transfer to the fetus. Drugs given intramuscularly lead to a more gradual rise and will reach a lower peak than the same dose given intravenously. It is important, therefore, to achieve the lowest level of drug in the maternal blood which is compatible with a therapeutic effect.

The size of the molecules of a substance is an important determinant of diffusion. Small molecules diffuse easily, while large molecules diffuse with difficulty or not at all. The majority of drugs have molecules of a size below the limit retarding diffusion, but some vital substances for the fetus, such as proteins, are too large to cross the placenta by diffusion. In this instance, the body has developed carriers which transport these substances across the placenta.

Glucose is a substance which crosses the placenta easily, but insulin, with its much larger molecules, cannot pass the placental barrier. In diabetics who become hypoglycaemic during labour, or even in normal patients given too much dextrose solution, the level of glucose in fetal blood rises to match that in maternal blood. The fetal hyperglycaemia stimulates the fetal pancreas to produce insulin. At delivery, the baby is cut off from the high glucose levels in the mother, but its own insulin level is still high, and this leads to dangerous hypoglycaemia. Hence the importance of keeping the blood sugar of diabetic mothers within the lower range of normal during labour, and of restricting the amount of dextrose solutions given to non-diabetic women.

Oxygen crosses the placenta by diffusion. The more oxygen given to the mother, the better the oxygenation of the fetus, although at oxygen levels beyond 60% there is a reduction in fetal oxygenation.

## Protein Binding

Not all of a drug in maternal blood is available for transfer to the fetus. This is because the majority of drugs are bound to a certain extent to plasma protein, and a drug bound to protein cannot cross the placenta; only the free, unbound drug is transferred. Hence, the greater the degree of protein binding, the less drug there is available for transfer. For instance, lignocaine is 50% bound and bupivicaine 95% bound, and they have F/M ratios of 0.7 and 0.3, respectively.

## Acidity

The degree of acidity in both maternal and fetal blood can affect the degree of placental transfer. The majority of drugs used in labour cross the placental barrier to a greater extent under acidic conditions. It is therefore important to avoid or treat acidosis (ketosis) in the mother.

## Placental Blood Flow

It is obvious that if there is no placental blood flow, then no drug will reach the fetus, but it also means that the fetus will die. During uterine contractions placental blood flow falls, and it is suggested that if an intravenous injection, for example, for induction of anaesthesia, is given during a uterine contraction, then highest maternal blood levels will be reached at a point when placental blood flow is reduced, so that transfer to the fetus will be less.

The measurement of the concentration of a drug in the umbilical vein does not necessarily indicate the response that may be expected. The level of drug in the umbilical artery, which is far more representative of the amount of drug being offered to, say, the fetal brain, is often lower than that in the umbilical vein. This is because a significant percentage of the umbilical venous blood perfuses the liver  before joining the systemic circulation. During its passage through the liver some of the drug may be removed. However, the ability of the fetus or newborn to break down drugs in the liver is limited because of deficiency or immaturity of the enzymes which perform this task. Furthermore, the ability to excrete drugs via the kidney is limited. In general, therefore, drugs gaining access to the fetus tend to remain in the tissues for a longer time than they do in an adult.

The possible effects on a fetus of drugs given to the mother are difficult to predict because of the variety of factors involved. The condition of the infant at birth will be further affected by obstetric factors. The baby's condition at birth is assessed by means of the Apgar score, a useful but still rather crude measurement, and limited by the fact that it is used only in the immediate period following delivery. This means that the more subtle and slowly developing effects of drugs used in labour may easily be missed. There has recently been much interest shown in these effects. Such factors as frequency of sucking, peak pressure developed during sucking and milk consumption are studied, together with a series of so-called neurobehavioural tests. These include:
    response to light
    response to sound
    primitive reflexes, such as the Moro reflex
    cuddliness
    consolability

Results of such studies have shown that the baby of a mother who has received one dose of pethidine in labour shows an overall decreased sucking ability, i.e. decreased sucking frequency, decreased peak sucking pressure, and therefore decreased overall milk consumption, when compared with the baby whose mother has received no drugs, or epidural analgesia. The same baby would be likely to show worse scores on the other tests listed above. These effects last for up to 48 hours. The significance of these effects is still a matter of conjecture,

**SUGGESTED FURTHER READING**

Corke, B.C. (1977) Neurobehavioural responses of the newborn: the effect of different forms of maternal analgesia. *Anaesthesia* 32:539.
Crawford, J. S. (1978) *Principles and Practice of Obstetric Anaesthesia,* 4th edn. Oxford: Blackwell Scientific Publications.

Green, J. H. (1969) *Basic Clinical Physiology.* London: Oxford Medical Publications.

Moir, D. D. (1980) *Obstetric Anaesthesia and Analgesia,* 2nd edn. London: Baillière Tindall.

Moir, D. D (1982) *Pain Relief in Labour,* 4th edn. Edinburgh: Churchill Livingstone.

Sweet, B. R. (1982) *Mayes' Midwifery — A Textbook for Midwives,* 1st edn. London: Baillière Tindall.

# 5 Requirements in Obstetric Anaesthesia

Because anaesthesia in obstetrics is a specialized area with its own particular problems there are certain requirements which will be considered under three headings:
Prevention of Mendelson's syndrome
Lack of maternal awareness
Minimal depression of the infant

**Prevention of Mendelson's Syndrome**
This is considered in some detail in Chapters 7 and 8. Mendelson's or acid aspiration syndrome is still a major cause of maternal mortality and morbidity in obstetric patients receiving general anaesthesia. Measures to prevent it include:
antacid therapy,
possibly emptying the stomach,
the use of cricoid pressure, and
endotracheal intubation

These measures are implemented on any pregnant patient from the second trimester until 24–48 hours after delivery. The increased use of regional techniques will also tend to reduce the incidence of Mendelson's syndrome.

**Lack of Maternal Awareness**
This requirement is closely linked with that of minimal depression of the infant, and is one of the fine balances which the obstetric anaesthetist is challenged to find.

Because of the risk of acid aspiration syndrome, the patient undergoing general anaesthesia for caesarean section will usually have an endotracheal tube inserted. Before endotracheal intubation can be carried out, reflex responses must be abolished. This may be done by inducing deep anaesthesia or by giving a muscle relaxant following induction of anaesthesia, so paralysing the patient. The former is not a suitable technique since all anaesthetic agents cross the placental barrier to some extent, and thus the latter approach is used. Because minimal anaesthesia is given prior to delivery of the baby, the patient's level of anaesthesia may become unacceptably light when the effect of the induction agent has worn off and her anaesthetic is being maintained by the inhalational agents, so that she becomes aware. However, because she has been paralysed by the use of a long-acting muscle relaxant to ensure toleration of the endotracheal tube, she will be unable to communicate that she is conscious. Studies indicate, however, that as few as 10% of patients who are thought to have been aware during anaesthesia have been able to recall any pain. Some patients will report nightmares, and this is thought to be due to subliminal awareness. Others will recall accurate snippets of conversation. Hearing is the last sensory perception to be lost in any state of unconsciousness, and the first to return, so that the use of earplugs, or headphones playing soothing music, may be helpful! Various studies have been carried out on this phenomenon, however, and anaesthetists are very aware of the problem, so that hopefully it now occurs much less frequently. The incidence of awareness when a thiopentone, nitrous oxide/oxygen and relaxant technique is used has been quoted as ranging from 8 to 42%. Supplementing nitrous oxide/oxygen with halothane reduces awareness very significantly to as little as 0.2%. Once the baby is delivered, the anaesthetic level can be deepened, and at this stage one of the morphine derivatives, such as fentanyl or phenoperidine, may be given intravenously; these give good analgesia and are commonly used.

If a patient does describe awareness, it is useful to inform the anaesthetist concerned. Occasionally a patient may be extremely distressed by this, particularly if she had expressed the frequently heard wish to be 'put out' so that she would know nothing of what went on. She may need to discuss the experience at length, and explanation and reassurance must be given. Tidings of such events unfortunately tend to travel far and wide, and her fellow patients in the ward may need reassurance too.

**Minimal Depression of the Infant**
Most drugs crossing the blood–brain barrier and affecting the central nervous system will similarly cross the placental barrier to affect the fetus. For this reason the patient who is to undergo elective caesarean section will not receive a narcotic premedication as she might under

other circumstances. The ideal length of the I–D interval (length of time elapsing between INDUCTION of anaesthesia and DELIVERY of the infant) has been the subject of considerable study and debate. 'Induction' in this context must not be confused with induction of labour! I–D interval is a term which may also be used in referring to the time elapsing between artificial rupture of the membranes and delivery.

Levels of induction agent, such as thiopentone and methohexitone, appear to reach their peak in fetal blood after 2–3 minutes, tailing off thereafter. Maintenance agents — nitrous oxide and volatile agents such as halothane — appear in slightly less predictable levels, but do appear almost immediately. Only in very rare cases does suxamethonium cross the placental barrier in sufficient quantities to affect the fetus at all. The long-acting muscle relaxants also pass into the fetal circulation in clinically insignificant quantities. Generally speaking, there is little to be gained by a minimal I–D interval, except in cases of fetal distress. Indeed, too brief an I–D interval is likely to result in a baby born at the time when his serum contains maximum quantities of his mother's anaesthetic induction agent. Many anaesthetists feel that the asphyxiated babies at caesarean section in the past may have suffered from reduced placental circulation as a result of maternal hypotension, and that if aortocaval occlusion and maternal hypoxia are avoided immediately prior to and during anaesthesia, an I–D interval of 10–20 minutes may be perfectly acceptable in terms of fetal well-being.

Of more significance, however, is the U–D interval. This is defined as the time elapsing from incision of the myometrium until delivery of the baby. The condition of the baby is likely to deteriorate as the U–D interval becomes greater. Incision of the myometrium almost certainly affects uteroplacental blood flow and probably expedites placental separation. In the event of difficult delivery, the baby may gasp before delivery is completed, so inhaling amniotic fluid or blood. Some obstetricians deliberately perform artificial rupture of the membranes prior to caesarean section in an attempt to prevent this.

## SUGGESTED FURTHER READING

Crawford, J. S. (1971) Awareness during operative obstetrics under general anaesthesia. *British Journal of Anaesthesia* 43:179.

Crawford, J. S. (1982) *Obstetric Analgesia and Anaesthesia* (Current Reviews in Obstetrics and Gynaecology series), 1st edn. Edinburgh: Churchill Livingstone.

Crawford, J. S., Burton, M., and Davies, P. (1973) Anaesthesia for caesarean section: further refinements of a technique. *British Journal of Anaesthesia* 45:726.

Husemeyer, R. P., Davenport, H. T., and Rajasekaren, T. (1978) Cimetidine as a single oral dose for prophylaxis against Mendelson's syndrome. *Anaesthesia* 33:775.

Lahiri, S. K., Thomas, T. A., and Hodgson, R. M. H. (1973) Single dose antacid therapy for the prevention of Mendelson's syndrome. *British Journal of Anaesthesia* 34:306.

Moir, D. D. (1980) *Obstetric Anaesthesia and Analgesia,* 2nd edn. London: Baillière Tindall.

Sellick, R. A. (1961) Cricoid pressure to control regurgitation of stomach contents during induction of anaesthesia: preliminary communication. *Lancet* ii:404.

Turndorf, H., Rodis, I. D., and Clark, T. S. (1974) 'Silent' regurgitation during general anaesthesia. *Anaesthesia and Analgesia, Current Research* 53:700.

# 6 Typical Anaesthetic for Caesarean Section

The purpose of this chapter is to outline a typical anaesthetic for caesarean section. Obviously individual anaesthetists will have their own preferences, but basic premises remain the same, even though the actual drugs used may vary.

### Premedication

Depending on whether the operation is elective or an emergency, the patient may or may not receive a premedication. In the case of an elective caesarean section, premedication may be cimetidine 300 mg or ranitidine 150 mg orally the night before operation, together with the same dose repeated two hours pre-operatively, perhaps with atropine 0.5 mg or hyoscine 0.4 mg intramuscularly. Alternatively, an antacid, sodium citrate 15–30 ml, or mist. magnesium trisilicate 30 ml, perhaps with atropine or hyoscine half an hour pre-operatively, may be given.

In emergency caesarean section, an antacid will be given, and, depending on the time available, atropine or hyoscine may be given intramuscularly, or intravenously at the time of induction.

The main principle underlying premedication for caesarean section is to raise the pH of gastric contents, so as to minimize the effects of Mendelson's syndrome should acid aspiration occur (see Chapter 8). Cimetidine and ranitidine are anti-histamine drugs which specifically block the secretion of acid by the stomach. They take some time to have an effect, and do not alter the acidity of stomach contents already present, so are less useful in an emergency. The advantage of the antacids is that they neutralize stomach contents quickly. There is some evidence to suggest that sodium citrate mixes more effectively with stomach contents than does mist. magnesium trisilicate, and that its effect on the lungs is less harmful, should aspiration occur.

A second principle is to dry up secretions. Both atropine and hyoscine achieve this but reduce tone in the lower oesophageal sphincter, thus increasing the risk of regurgitation. Hyoscine reduces the incidence of maternal awareness during anaesthesia. A comparatively new drug, glycopyrrolate (Robinul), has the advantage of crossing the placenta to a lesser extent.

It has been shown that the baby's general condition at birth is better if the mother has been lying on her side for at least half an hour prior to general anaesthesia. She is therefore encouraged to lie on her side, often the right side if left lateral tilt is employed in the theatre, so as to facilitate mixing of the antacid with gastric contents.

**Pre-oxygenation**
The patient is pre-oxygenated, that is, she is given oxygen by face mask, prior to general anaesthesia. This improves both maternal and fetal $PO_2$, providing a safeguard in the event of any hypoxic episode, such as failed or difficult intubation (see Chapter 8). If the patient wishes, she may hold the mask for herself; she should be encouraged to hold it firmly in place so that no room air is inhaled. This ensures that she breathes pure oxygen. Pre-oxygenation is continued for at least three, and preferably five minutes, without interruption. At this stage, the patient will either be on the operating table, with 15° of left lateral tilt, or a trolley with a wedge or pillow under her right buttock, so that the gravid uterus is displaced laterally to prevent aortocaval occlusion. The facility to tip the patient head-down must be available. During pre-oxygenation, the anaesthetist will check his equipment — Boyles machine, laryngoscopes, endotracheal tubes and suction. He will also check that the patient's intravenous infusion is running well.

**Induction of Anaesthesia**
After pre-oxygenation, thiopentone 225 mg–275 mg, depending on the size of the patient, is injected, followed by suxamethonium (Scoline) 100 mg. During the injection of thiopentone, cricoid pressure is applied by the anaesthetist's assistant and is maintained until the cuff of the endotracheal tube is inflated and the seal is checked. As soon as fascicula-tion (generalized twitching of the muscles) occurs, indicating the onset of action of the suxamethonium, endotracheal intubation is performed. The cuff is inflated, the seal checked, and the chest auscultated to ascertain that both lungs are being ventilated. The tube is then secured with tape or strapping. One of the other induction agents such as methohexitone, althesin or etomidate may be used.

**Maintenance**

Once the endotracheal tube is in position, the patient is usually given 50% oxygen and 50% nitrous oxide (usually about four litres/minute of each), together with 0.5% halothane or 0.8%–1.0% enflurane, and connected to a ventilator. It is important that the patient is not hyperventilated, since this will lead to a fall in maternal $PCO_2$, with the result that maternal haemoglobin will retain oxygen and not release it for passage across the placenta.

The effect of the suxamethonium is normally short-lived (3–5 minutes) and, once this effect has worn off, muscle relaxation is maintained using alcuronium, curare or pancuronium.

*Before Delivery*

Prior to delivery of the baby, the anaesthetic action of nitrous oxide and oxygen is supplemented by halothane or enflurane in order to prevent maternal awareness. At the low concentrations already described, the effect of these two volatile agents on the uterus is negligible, but at higher concentrations they tend to cause relaxation of the uterus, resulting in an increased incidence of post-partum haemorrhage and intra-operative bleeding. Trichloroethylene (Trilene) may be used, but there is no doubt that it is associated with a higher incidence of maternal awareness.

*Following Delivery*

As soon as the baby's head is delivered, the anaesthetist will inject an oxytocic drug to contract the uterus; syntocinon, usually five units intravenously, is the preferred oxytocic. Occasionally ergometrine 0.5 mg may be given, but it should not be given to patients with pre-eclampsia or essential hypertension, since it tends to cause a sudden rise in blood pressure. Often the initial bolus dose of syntocinon is supplemented with 5–20 units of syntocinon in an intravenous infusion given over a period of 1–2 hours, in order to maintain contraction of the uterus. Once the umbilical cord has been clamped, anaesthesia is deepened by increasing the concentration of nitrous oxide to 60–70% and by giving an intravenous opiate, after which the volatile supplement is usually turned off. Any opiate may be used; those most commonly given are fentanyl 100–250 μg, phenoperidine 1.0–1.5 mg, pethidine 50 mg or papaveretum 10–20 mg. An anti-emetic such as perphenazine or droperidol may be given with the opiate.

## Reversal

At the end of the operation, the effects of the muscle relaxant are reversed by giving neostigmine 2.5 mg together with atropine. The latter is used to counteract undesirable side effects of neostigmine — bradycardia, increased salivary and bronchial secretions, and spasm of the gut. The anaesthetist may already have added some carbon dioxide to the anaesthetic gases in order to raise the level of carbon dioxide in the blood, thus stimulating the respiratory centre. The nitrous oxide is turned off, and the patient breathes oxygen. If spontaneous respiration appears to have been re-established, the patient is turned onto her side, pharyngeal suction is performed, the cuff of the endotracheal tube is deflated, and the tube is removed. The patient is transferred to her bed, still in the lateral position. Regurgitation and inhalation of stomach contents is still a distinct possibility in the post-operative period and the recovering patient must not be left unattended. Cough, cyanosis, wheezing and a fall in blood pressure are all indicative of possible acid aspiration, and the anaesthetist should be informed immediately if they occur.

Post-operative analgesia and fluid therapy will be prescribed by the anaesthetist before the patient leaves the theatre area. He may ask that the patient be given oxygen by face mask for a time in the recovery area.

## SUGGESTED FURTHER READING

Bonica, J. J. (1972) *Obstetric Analgesia and Anesthesia.* Berlin: Springer-Verlag.

Crawford, J. S. (1971) Awareness during operative obstetrics under general anaesthesia. *British Journal of Anaesthesia* 43:179.

Crawford, J. S. (1978) *Principles and Practice of Obstetric Anaesthesia,* 4th edn. Oxford: Blackwell Scientific Publications.

Crawford, J. S., Burton, M., and Davies, P. (1973) Anaesthesia for Caesarean section: further refinements of a technique. *British Journal of Anaesthesia* 45:726.

Moir, D. D. (1980) *Obstetric Anaesthesia and Analgesia,* 2nd edn. London: Baillière Tindall.

# 7 *Nursing Responsibilities*

## INTRODUCTION

The nursing process is currently the subject of much debate. There are problems associated with its use in midwifery, though the underlying principles are a good basis for giving nursing care. The care of every patient in the labour room as well as during the post-natal period may certainly be considered by using a 'problem solving' approach. By analysis of each individual situation and identification of potential problems, it should be possible to improve patient care in the labour ward suite. This is already being done, of course, and the patient with a possible cephalopelvic disproportion, or one who has had an ante-partum haemorrhage or a malpresentation, will be treated as one who may require general anaesthesia at any stage. However, there is scope for this 'problem identification' approach to be applied in the ante-natal period. At the present time, this problem identification may be limited to a cryptic entry by a doctor in the patient's notes, such as 'may need C.S.'. The patient may be unaware of this, so that a potential obstetric problem has been identified but nothing more has been done. From this potential obstetric problem various potential midwifery problems may be elicited. The role of the midwife in the ante-natal period has become a rather less active one in recent years, but this pattern will undoubtedly change, partly as a result of pressure from the midwives themselves, and perhaps also as a result of public opinion and consumer demand. Whenever midwives are able to run their own ante-natal clinics, ideally seeing the same patients, so that a relationship is established and the patient thinks of a particular midwife as 'her' midwife, the nursing process may be implemented from an early stage. Even without this rather idealistic 'one to one' relationship, the nursing process has obvious advantages for both the midwife and her patients. Perhaps the greatest of these advantages is that continuity of care and the giving of consistent advice may be facilitated, using the nursing process. Innumerable women have suffered confusion and total loss of self-confidence (as well as loss of confidence in those caring for them) at a time when they are emotionally very vulnerable, as the result of conflicting advice given by conscientious, caring individuals. The classic example is probably the establishment and management of breast feeding.

The nursing process is described as:

*Assessment.* At this stage, problems, potential problems or needs of a physical, psychological/emotional or social nature are identified and noted.

*Planning nursing care.* Goals related to the identified problems or needs are now defined and noted.

*Implementing nursing care.* All nursing care given in the attempt to meet the defined needs is recorded on the Nursing Care Plan. A mental evaluation is made as this is done, even though the formal evaluation comes later.

*Evaluating nursing care.* Goals are examined and reviewed at suitable intervals. This means that nursing care becomes meaningful and is tailored to the needs of the individual patient. Tradition and routine need no longer be carried out in a mechanical fashion.

This gives patient-orientated care and is therefore satisfying. Patient allocation rather than task allocation is almost certain to improve standards of patient care and to help the professionals to see the individual patient and her particular situation as a whole and to view it realistically.

Now, more than ever before, the media and the public are placing a lot of emphasis on alternative methods of childbirth and on women's rights of choice. The nursing process lends itself as a means of improving continuity of care, communication, patient involvement, and many other areas commonly criticized in the maternity services. In some centres, women at the ante-natal clinic are encouraged to consider and discuss their preferences, for example, their position for delivery, whether or not they wish to put the baby to the breast immediately, and their views on analgesia. These preferences are commonly recorded on a 'Birth Plan' which is filed in the mother's notes. A 'Birth Plan' is not unlike a 'Nursing Care Plan', and it facilitates the identification of midwifery objectives or problems as opposed to obstetric problems. There will always be patients who will not wish to be so actively involved in their care and who will feel that the professionals are there to make the decisions. However, many will welcome the opportunity to make informed decisions regarding the management of their own pregnancy and labour.

While, as already indicated, the identification of obstetric problems or potential problems may highlight areas of interest to the midwife, many midwifery objectives are identified quite independently. The midwife is not required to concern herself with those areas dealt with by the obstetrician or general practitioner, but has a vast, even daunting scope in discussing diet, minor ailments and discomforts in pregnancy, sources of worry such as the care of other children, and financial or housing problems. More specifically, discussion with the multiparous woman on the subject of her previous labours, analgesia and deliveries, may help her to clarify her feelings regarding her requirements in her current pregnancy and anticipated labour.

It is here, too, that the opportunity presents itself to prepare the patient for possible eventualities, whenever this seems appropriate, for example, when caesarean section seems likely. Giving a woman time to accept and consider the possibilities will often make her feel better prepared and less anxious. She has time to discuss her apprehension and ask her questions; here too is the opportunity for labour ward or theatre staff to meet her, so that she may anticipate seeing someone who is not a complete stranger when she has her baby. Ante-natal classes have long played their part in this preparation, but the value of 'one to one' contact should not be underestimated.

'Nursing care plans' are used for documentation of the nursing process, and they are designed to meet the needs of any particular area or speciality of nursing. Care plans in midwifery would ideally go to the community midwife and then to the health visitor, where of course the nursing process is equally useful. In discussing nursing responsibilities with regard to the patient about to undergo general anaesthesia, it will be assumed that the reader is familiar with the procedure for preparation of the patient for theatre which is in use in his or her own hospital. The following discussion is therefore not intended to deal comprehensively with such procedures, but to pick out certain salient points.

## THE PRE-OPERATIVE PERIOD

### Preparation of the Patient

*Psychological.* While some obstetric patients will be receiving anaesthesia for elective procedures, many will be about to undergo surgery in an emergency situation, often one fraught with a sense of considerable urgency, the concern usually being with regard to the fetus rather than the mother. In such instances the patient will have become aware of the urgency, and her anxiety for her baby adds to the distress she was already feeling. She may well have been in established labour for some time and may therefore feel exhausted. Opiate or inhalational analgesia, or both, may have dimmed her awareness of fact and fiction and her perception of time, and the inevitable flurry of activity which precedes an emergency caesarean section must often become a nightmare for such a patient. However, preparation procedures must be carried out, and with as little time wasted as possible. Positive support and encouragement of these patients, giving realistic reassurance and as much explanation as the individual patient requires, is a demanding challenge recognized by all midwives. The patient may feel a profound sense of failure at having been unable to deliver spontaneously, however sensitively she may have been prepared for labour. Again, many of these women will feel deeply disappointed at not being able to participate in delivery if circumstances are such that caesarean section under epidural block is not feasible. Their anxieties with regard to bonding and their husband's welfare must be sensed, and reassurance given, when possible. There can be no doubt in any quarter as to the positive value of care by one midwife throughout labour, particularly once a relationship and effective communication have been established. If this midwife can prepare her patient for theatre, remain with her during induction of anaesthesia and care for her during the recovery period, then one source of stress — a series of new faces — must have been reduced for the patient.

Many anxieties will arise as to the anaesthetic procedure, the recovery period, the effects of the anaesthetic on the baby and on the successful establishment of breast feeding. For some patients there may be anxiety about the possibility or number of future pregnancies. Language difficulties will be another factor in many such cases (an 'index' of volunteer interpreters for various languages may be available, and this can be invaluable). These are the kinds of anxieties voiced by women who are to undergo elective procedures, perhaps more so than by those in an emergency situation, since these women will have had more time to ponder long-term consequences.

*Physical.* Physical preparation will not be discussed in fine detail, since this will vary from one centre to another. Antacid regimes throughout labour are currently in vogue, and the giving of antacids once general anaesthesia is a certainty is of prime importance. The woman in labour is usually permitted fluids only by mouth, although, in the occasional emergency situation, the patient may have eaten prior to admission (see Chapter 5). The bladder should be empty; a catheter is often inserted. The presence of crowns, bridges, caps and loose teeth should be clearly recorded on the notes, and the nurse should ensure that the anaesthetist is aware of this information so that he can avoid spoiling the dentist's handiwork during intubation. Dentures, contact lenses and make-up, including nail varnish, should be removed. Jewellery is usually covered and any valuables are placed in safe-keeping.

The patient's identity and proposed operation must be verbally checked, preferably with the patient herself, but with another nurse if the patient is unconscious or very distressed. Identification bands and notes must be cross-checked at the same time. Written consent to surgery should have been obtained, and this is also checked. Blood will usually have been cross-matched; on occasions surgery is delayed until it is actually available.

**Preparation of Equipment**
Anaesthetic equipment must be checked before use, and while the anaesthetist will certainly carry out his own check before proceeding to give an anaesthetic, a double check is undoubtedly more satisfactory.

*The Boyles machine.* The anaesthetist's assistant must be sufficiently familiar with the Boyles machine to be able to carry out basic checking procedures. Of prime importance are the gas supply and the suction apparatus. The piped supply must be connected, or the cylinders open, as applicable. If a piped supply is present, cylinders must be checked in case of failure of the primary supply, but should then be left closed. Each flowmeter in turn must be checked for gas flow; the bobbin should rise to the top of the gauge when turned full on; it should spin, and then sink when the gas supply is turned off. Only the appropriate bobbin should rise when any one gas is being tested. The emergency oxygen flush should be operated briefly and at the same time the patency of the black reservoir bag on the Magill circuit checked; the circuit itself should be seen to be complete and correctly assembled. A quick glance at the vaporizers should be sufficient to ascertain that a fluid level is visible in each port-hole.

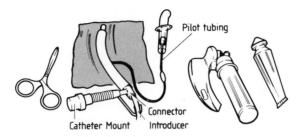

**Fig. 7.1** Equipment for endotracheal intubation. A typical layout of equipment ready for endotracheal intubation — from left to right: Artery forceps, a cuffed oral endotracheal tube and introducer, a laryngoscope, and lubricant jelly.

*Intubation equipment* (Fig. 7.1). The laryngoscope should give a bright, consistent light, and a spare one should be readily available and in good working order. Points to check if the laryngoscope does not function well are batteries, bulbs and contacts. Supplies of batteries and bulbs should be kept in the theatre area; the contacts may require cleaning with a spirit swab. If cleaning the contacts does not help, it may simply be that the screw holding the spring-clip needs to be tightened (this applies to the screw-type handle). If none of these simple measures is effective, the laryngoscope must be sent to the appropriate department for repair.

*Endotracheal tubes.* The correct size must be available and a full range of tubes must be readily to hand. Endotracheal tubes must be of suitable length; too long a tube may enter the right main bronchus so that only one lung is inflated, while too short a tube may not adequately protect the airway. A cuffed endotracheal tube requires a 10 ml syringe for inflating the cuff and a pair of artery forceps with which to clamp the tubing from the cuff so as to keep it inflated. The cuff and its pilot balloon should be inflated and checked before use. The following must also be ready for use:
   gauze swabs
   lubricant
   Magill's introducing forceps
   airways
   face mask
   suction ends and catheters

mouth gag
tongue forceps
spatula
tape to secure the tube in position

The intubation equipment is laid out so that it is readily accessible. Immediately prior to induction of anaesthesia, the suction equipment is turned on and the sucker is placed by the patient's head, for example, under the pillow. As the assistant is not free to move away from the patient, it is conveniently placed there for immediate use.

The equipment necessary for an intravenous infusion must be prepared, and monitoring equipment should be ready for use. The anaesthetist will measure the patient's blood pressure at regular intervals; he may monitor pulse rate and cardiac rhythm by the use of an ECG giving an oscilloscope display. A pre-eclamptic patient, or one who is shocked following, for example, a severe ante-partum haemorrhage, may have had central venous and arterial lines inserted, so that central venous and arterial pressures may be monitored.

### Reception of the Patient
The patient's fears and anxieties have already been discussed, and she will need sympathetic support and encouragement until the moment she is anaesthetized. It is common for patients about to have a caesarean section to be anaesthetized in the operating theatre rather than in the anaesthetic room, and many patients will feel even more apprehensive at this thought. Again, reassurance and some explanation will be required, and background noise and activity must be kept to a minimum. As few people as possible should be round the patient before induction of anaesthesia. She will not have had the advantage of a sedative premedication because of the likelihood of depressing the fetus, and so may be very aware of all that is happening.

If the nurse from the labour ward hands the patient into the care of another nurse in the anaesthetic room, all details of identity and proposed operation must be checked, and all relevant information given.

## DURING ANAESTHESIA

### Positioning of the Patient
There is always a danger of injury to the unconscious patient unless

meticulous care is taken to position her safely. The main point to consider is the position of limbs and head. The limbs must be secured in a position comfortable to the patient and convenient to the anaesthetist and surgeon before induction of anaesthesia. Pressure on calves, ankles and elbows must be avoided, and where arms are secured on an arm board, adduction of the arm beyond 90° must also be avoided. Damage to nerve plexuses and transient or longer-term dysfunction may result from lack of attention to such detail. Pressure on calves may increase the likelihood of deep vein thrombosis in the puerperium.

The patient's head must be completely supported by the stretcher canvas. She will lift her own head whilst conscious, and inadequate support may not be noticed until she is lifted again, when injury to the neck could result. No part of the patient must be in contact with any metal, since this may result in electrical burns if diathermy is used.

The full supine position must be avoided to prevent hypotension due to aortocaval occlusion. The use of a wedge under the buttocks or of lateral tilt of the operating table will displace the gravid uterus to one side and prevent pressure on the great vessels.

The anaesthetist's assistant must be familiar with the operation of the theatre table and the use of all fittings, so that it is used with complete safety and versatility.

Care must be taken in positioning the patient to prevent displacement of intravenous infusions or catheter.

## Assisting the Anaesthetist

If the midwife finds herself assisting the anaesthetist she must be sure that she understands the principles involved in obstetric anaesthesia, and must seek instruction where necessary. She must familiarize herself with the layout of the theatre and with emergency procedures.

### Cricoid Pressure

One of the most vital procedures which the anaesthetic assistant must perform is cricoid pressure. The Report on Confidential Enquiries into Maternal Deaths (in England and Wales, 1973–75) describes several cases of Mendelson's syndrome which could have been prevented by efficient application of cricoid pressure. The investigators then said: 'Cricoid pressure is a matter for a skilled and practised assistant to the anaesthetist, not for casual delegation to others.' Cricoid pressure is a procedure designed to protect the airway from regurgitated stomach contents.

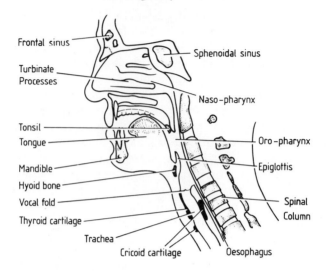

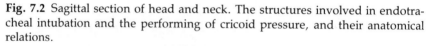

**Fig. 7.2** Sagittal section of head and neck. The structures involved in endotracheal intubation and the performing of cricoid pressure, and their anatomical relations.

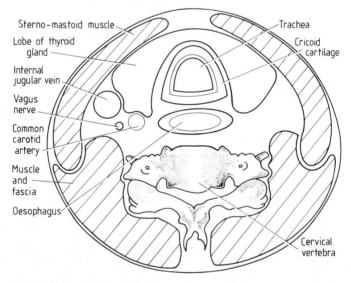

**Fig. 7.3** The structures of the neck. This diagrammatic cross-section at the level of the 6th cervical vertebra (C6) shows the anatomical relations of the cricoid cartilage.

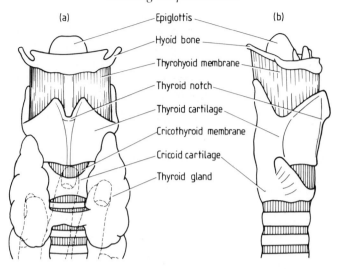

(a)          Epiglottis        (b)

Hyoid bone

Thyrohyoid membrane

Thyroid notch

Thyroid cartilage

Cricothyroid membrane

Cricoid cartilage

Thyroid gland

**Fig. 7.4** Sellick's manoeuvre. This diagrammatic representation of one method of performing cricoid pressure shows the underlying anatomical structures. (a) Front view, (b) lateral view.

It utilizes the cricoid cartilage (Fig. 7.2), which is a complete ring of cartilage around the trachea (Fig. 7.3), to occlude the oesophagus (Fig. 7.4) by applying steady pressure towards the cervical spine.

The cricoid cartilage is identified by careful palpation, starting at the sternal notch. With the patient's head extended, it is usually the first cartilaginous prominence encountered. If pressure is applied too high, at the level of the thyroid cartilage or 'Adam's apple', occlusion of the oesophagus will be incomplete, partly because the thyroid cartilage is not a complete ring of cartilage and partly because this point is almost at the level of the oropharynx where the oesophagus and trachea originate. Pressure at this point will also tend to partly occlude the cords, thus impeding intubation.

Sellick described cricoid pressure as an efficient means of preventing Mendelson's syndrome in 1961, and one method of performing cricoid pressure now bears his name. In Sellick's manoeuvre, the cricoid cartilage is located and, using the thumb and second finger to steady the trachea in the midline (Fig. 7.4), firm pressure is applied on the cricoid cartilage using the index finger. The patient will find this procedure unpleasant if it is performed before or at the start of induction of anaesthesia, particularly since she will tend to feel a heightened awareness of sound and touch immediately before hypnosis occurs. The assistant should explain her actions to the patient, and then define the cricoid cartilage and position her fingers lightly. As the patient loses consciousness and prior to administration of the muscle relaxant, the cricoid pressure should be steadily applied. The pressure must be maintained until the endotracheal tube is in position and its cuff is both inflated and checked. If in any doubt, the assistant must ask the anaesthetist's permission before releasing the pressure. In the event of difficulty with intubation and failure to pass the endotracheal tube, it may be necessary to maintain cricoid pressure throughout the anaesthetic. In this instance care must be taken to provide cricoid pressure only; too zealous an application of pressure could cause a degree of venous congestion as a result of indirect pressure on the internal jugular veins.

Some anaesthetists may prefer a slightly different technique, but the principles remain the same. If the patient should vomit (rather than regurgitate) while cricoid pressure is being applied, it is usual to release the pressure, since oesophageal rupture is a real danger. The anaesthetist will make this decision.

**Coping with Emergencies**

*Difficult Intubation (see also Chapter 8)*
Difficulty with intubation may be anticipated if the patient has any physical problems such as limitation of movement of the jaw or cervical spine, any abnormalities of neck or throat, or any relevant medical history. However, such difficulty may arise quite unexpectedly with any patient. It may be associated with laryngeal oedema, which may be seen in pregnant women at term, especially those with pre-eclampsia. Failure to pass an endotracheal tube at the first attempt will lead to local trauma and increased oedema.

The assistant's responsibilities include being familiar with the local procedure and anticipating the anaesthetist's needs. She will not be able to leave the patient if she is maintaining cricoid pressure, but she may need to delegate to others and to call for further medical and nursing assistance if necessary. There will be a 'runner' or circulating nurse in the theatre, and she must be given an accurate, succinct message and clear instructions, if sent to summon help.

## Haemorrhage

The patient who has suffered an ante-partum or post-partum haemorrhage may be profoundly shocked. Blood loss will need to be assessed and replaced as accurately as possible. Blood or other fluids may need to be given quickly; a pressure infusion bag, such as the Fenwal bag, may be used for this. Accurate fluid balance records must be kept. Equipment for warming blood should be available, and the midwife should be familiar with its use. The blood warmer is thermostatically controlled to heat water to a certain temperature. A blood warming coil is incorporated into the intravenous line so that the cold blood runs through the coil, which is immersed in the water. This raises the blood to approximately body temperature before it is transfused. Equipment for central venous pressure and arterial lines must be available. The midwife will need to observe and record any further blood loss and any change in the patient's condition.

## Cardiac Arrest

Hypotension and hypoxia are problems which must be prevented whenever possible. However, should they occur together the outcome may well be cardiac arrest. If this occurs in the theatre area the usual first aid measures with, for example, a Brook airway or Ambu bag will probably not be required. A good airway will usually have been established, except where cardiac arrest has occurred as the result of failure to intubate the trachea. In this case desperate measures are needed, and some form of tracheotomy, such as cricothyroid puncture, and insertion of some means of giving oxygen may be necessary. If the patient's lungs can be inflated and oxygenated, the assistant can usefully commence external cardiac massage.

External cardiac massage is a skill which needs to be maintained. It will rarely be used in an obstetric unit, but the midwife needs to feel confident that she can perform it if necessary. It is very much a first aid measure, but the first few moments of cardiac arrest are critical, and restoration of some kind of cardiac function is essential. The patient should be on a hard surface, preferably the floor, for the benefit of the person performing cardiac massage, since he or she will find it arduous, tiring work after a very short period, and it will be ineffective, wasted effort if performed on a subject lying on a mattress. The stimulus to the heart is provided by repeated intermittent pressure from the lower third of the sternum. The operator places the 'heel' of one hand on the centre of the lower third of the sternum, with the 'heel' of the other hand on top; keeping the elbows straight to prevent wasted effort, he then exerts and releases a rapid downwards pressure. This is repeated at the rate of a normal pulse, that is, about 70 compressions per minute.

In the absence of other skilled assistance, the person performing the cardiac massage would also have to inflate the patient's lungs, using either mouth-to-mouth or mouth-to-nose ventilation. This is extremely arduous! An appropriate rhythm for resuscitation is five cardiac compressions followed by one inflation of the lungs, and it is useful to count aloud. An ECG and defibrillator should be available, and a tray of emergency drugs should be ready for use at all times. Emergency drugs will include:

**Adrenaline.** Used in doses of 0.5–10 ml of a 1:10 000 solution (adrenaline is supplied in ampoules containing 1:1 000 strength). It is injected intravenously to:

convert asystole to fibrillation,

convert fine fibrillation to coarse fibrillation,

raise the blood pressure.

Doses can be repeated as required.

**Atropine.** May be used to treat asystole or sinus bradycardia.

**Lignocaine.** Given when ventricular fibrillation or ventricular tachycardia does not respond to defibrillation. A bolus dose of 50–100 mg intravenously is used.

**Bretylium.** Another drug used if ventricular fibrillation or ventricular tachycardia is resistant to defibrillation.

**Calcium gluconate.** Of limited usefulness, but may be used in cardiovascular collapse due to haemorrhage, for example.

**Sodium bicarbonate.** Used to correct the metabolic acidosis which occurs following tissue hypoxia. It must be used alongside effective ventilation and oxygenation. Prompt, effective cardiopulmonary resuscitation will often obviate the need to use sodium bicarbonate.

**Isoprenaline.** May be indicated to treat the bradycardia due to heart block. It is a temporary measure used until a pace-maker can be inserted.

A variety of other drugs may be required and must be available for emergency use, but they are relevant to the underlying cause of the cardiac arrest and are not primarily involved in restoring cardiac function. They include:

Frusemide
Heparin
Aminophylline
Hydrocortisone
50% Dextrose

The principles in the treatment of cardiac arrest are:
i) to establish and maintain an airway
ii) to reverse hypoxia and metabolic acidosis
iii) to restore adequate cardiac output, initially by the first aid measure of external cardiac massage, and subsequently by improving myocardial tone and regulating myocardial activity by use of drugs and defibrillation
iv) to raise the blood pressure
v) to treat the cause if possible
vi) to monitor progress by continuous ECG recording, arterial blood gas estimation and chest X-rays.

Arterial blood gas analysis gives the most reliable guide to the degree of hypoxia and hypercapnia, and the progress of treatment. An arterial line gives a more satisfactory means of access to arterial blood than repeated arterial puncture. It is usually more appropriate for the obstetric patient who has suffered cardiac arrest to be nursed in an Intensive Therapy Unit rather than in the Obstetric Unit, and she is likely to be transferred there when her condition allows.

**Assistance at Extubation**
Assistance at extubation is as important as assistance at intubation. Once the endotracheal tube has been removed, the danger of inhalation of regurgitated stomach contents is still present until the patient has recovered full consciousness. It is true that the endotracheal tube is not removed until the patient shows signs of objecting to its presence, in other words, when her reflexes have returned. However, silent regurgitation may still occur and because she is drowsy, the patient may inhale vomitus. The assistant must therefore be on hand for extubation and must give help with suction, the giving of oxygen, with providing head-down tilt of the operating table or positioning the patient on her side as necessary.

## THE RECOVERY PERIOD

### Care of the Unconscious Patient

The positioning of the patient post-operatively is as important as it is in the pre-operative period, though the emphasis is different. The recovering patient may be restless and may move suddenly. She must be supported securely on her side, and again care must be taken of limbs, the intravenous infusion, the catheter, and wound drainage bottles. The most important point is to prevent obstruction of the airway, though this is less likely to occur if the patient is on her side.

The semi-prone position is sometimes referred to as the recovery position. It allows drainage of secretions from the mouth and prevents airway obstruction by the tongue. The patient is secure in this position even if she tends to be restless, and the dressing is quite easily observed. If the patient is nursed in the supine position, airway obstruction by the tongue is prevented by lifting the jaw forwards and upwards. Obstetric patients are usually safer recovering in the lateral position, though this will depend on circumstances, for not all pregnant women undergoing surgery will be operated on for obstetric reasons. Every nurse caring for a patient recovering from general anaesthesia must be alert for the signs of an obstructed airway and must be able to treat this problem promptly and efficiently. Noisy breathing almost always indicates a degree of airway obstruction, but airway obstruction does not always cause noisy breathing. Lifting the jaw forwards and upwards will usually relieve airway obstruction by the tongue, and the patient's jaw may need to be supported in this position until she regains full consciousness. The patient may leave the operating theatre with an oral airway in position. This may be removed, often by the patient herself, as soon as she has recovered sufficiently to object to its presence. An airway should be reinserted in the recovering patient with caution and only if it is really necessary, since it may stimulate vomiting.

Wherever the post-operative patient is nursed, certain basic facilities must be available. These are:

Suction

Oxygen

A good light to allow observation of the patient's colour

Beds or trolleys of a height and width suitable to nursing needs. Trolleys must be provided with cot sides, and both beds and trolleys must include 'head-down' tilt. They must be easily manoeuvred and steered.

An emergency call system, and ideally also a telephone

Emergency resuscitation equipment, including an Ambu bag or similar resuscitation bag, intubation equipment and a tray of emergency drugs.

## Observations and Monitoring

The patient's general condition — appearance, particularly colour, and level of consciousness — should be noted and recorded as soon as she reaches the recovery area, and all dressings and drains and the urinary catheter, if present, should be inspected. The uterine fundus is palpated; it should remain firm, and the lochia should also be observed. Her temperature, pulse and blood pressure should then be measured and recorded. The intravenous infusion site should also be inspected, and the functioning of the infusion itself should be checked. If the patient is passing from the care of one nurse to another, all relevant details of surgery and anaesthesia, and post-operative orders must be passed on. The anaesthetist may ask for oxygen to be given by face mask for a time.

Blood pressure and pulse are recorded as frequently as the patient's condition indicates or in accordance with medical orders. Respiration (patency of the airway) and colour are also observed and recorded. Post-operative analgesia is given as soon as necessary. If such analgesia proves inadequate and the patient remains distressed, the anaesthetist should be informed. If an epidural catheter remains in position after the patient's labour, very satisfactory post-operative analgesia may be provided via this route.

The baby also needs to be observed during the period in the recovery area.

## THE PATIENT REQUIRING INTENSIVE CARE

Intensive care in obstetrics is required for severe pre-eclampsia or eclampsia or for the patient who has suffered severe ante-partum or post-partum haemorrhage. The unstable diabetic will need careful nursing following delivery, particularly if delivered by caesarean section. The patient with any underlying disease or physical disability may also require intensive care and a 'special' nurse.

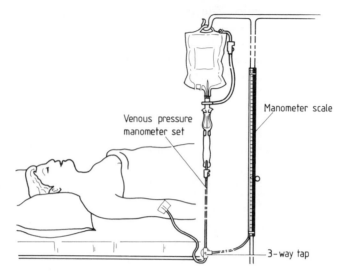

Venous pressure
manometer set

Manometer scale

3-way tap

**Fig. 7.5** A central venous pressure line.


**Central Venous Pressure Lines**
Central venous pressure (CVP) lines are now frequently used in general
wards as a guide to the patient's circulatory function in terms of cardiac
output and circulatory volume. Central venous pressure is equivalent
to pressure in the right atrium, and gives good indication as to whether
the patient is hypovolaemic or is being over-transfused. In obstetric
patients, a cannula is usually passed via a distal site, such as an ante-
cubital vein, into the superior vena cava. In other patients the subclavian
or internal jugular vein may be used. There is a risk of pneumothorax
occurring when these more central entry sites are used. A chest X-ray
is usually performed to confirm the position of the venous catheter.

Measurement of central venous pressure may be made via a transducer
onto monitoring equipment, or by means of a water manometer giving
a reading in centimetres of water (cm $H_2O$) (Fig. 7.5).

*Equipment*
In the latter instance, the following equipment will be needed:
   A venous pressure manometer set, primed with clear fluid such as
   Hartmanns solution
   An adjustable drip stand complete with the special manometer scale

A selection of central venous lines
A sterile basic towel set, plus gown and gloves
Solution or spray for cleaning the skin
Local anaesthetic, syringe and needle
A selection of dressings and strapping
A spirit level
An indelible skin marker

*Procedure*

The skin is cleaned using aseptic technique. The operator will normally wear a sterile gown and gloves. A tourniquet is used and the vein located. The skin is anaesthetized and the line primed and inserted. Central venous line 'sets' include a cannula and various devices designed to facilitate 'non-touch technique'. The entry site may be sprayed with an iodine or antibiotic spray, and a sterile dressing is applied. The line is securely fixed in place, and attached to the venous pressure manometer set.

The central venous line may be used as a 'main line' for infusion of clear fluids as well as for a venous manometer. The manometer line is taped to the manometer scale on the drip stand in such a way that it can be adjusted. A three-way tap is included in the 'venous pressure manometer set' to open the line to the infusion or to the manometer. The pressure should always be read having estimated 'zero' from the same point. This is commonly the point on the mid-axillary line which lies nearest the midpoint of the sternum; this is at the level of the right atrium. Clear and accurate marking of this 'mid-axillary point' will allow accurate readings of central venous pressure, since its relation to the right atrium does not vary with changes in the patient's position. It is marked on the skin, using the indelible marker. The spirit level is then used to place the 'zero' point on the manometer scale exactly level with this point (Fig. 7.6). The reading may then be taken by allowing fluid to run into the manometer line and then closing the line to the infusion, that is, 'opening' it to the patient and the manometer. The fluid level in the manometer will now settle at central venous pressure, and the fluid level will be seen to fluctuate slightly with the patient's respirations. The mean of the fluctuation levels may be read as central venous pressure; normal readings are between 3 and 10 cm $H_2O$, though they are higher during artificial ventilation. A lower reading suggests hypovolaemia, while a higher reading may indicate over-transfusion or right-sided heart failure.

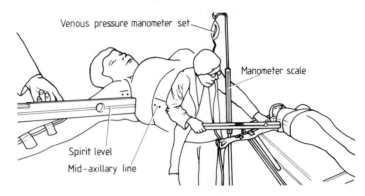

Venous pressure manometer set

Manometer scale

Spirit level

Mid–axillary line

**Fig. 7.6** Measuring central venous pressure. This diagram shows the marking of the mid-axillary line and the mid-axillary point, and the use of a spirit level to determine 'zero' in order to give consistently accurate readings of central venous pressure.

*Complications*

*Infection.* This risk is obviously increased if the CVP line remains in place for a period of days. The entry site should be re-dressed and sprayed with antibiotic spray regularly. Careful aseptic technique at insertion is vitally important.

*Thrombo-phlebitis.* This is more likely to occur when a peripheral line is used.

*Pneumothorax.* This is a complication seen with a subclavian or internal jugular line. Haemothorax or haematoma of the neck may also occur.

*Blockage of the CVP line.* A continual flow of fluid through the CVP line, even a very slow flow, will prevent blockage of the line by clot formation. Clot formation may result in an embolism.

**Arterial Lines**

Arterial cannulation is performed for two main reasons:
Measurement of arterial blood pressure
Access to arterial blood samples for blood gas estimation

Measurement of arterial blood pressure is performed via a transducer onto an electronic monitoring device.

*Equipment*

Equipment required includes:

The same basic towel set as for insertion of a central venous pressure line, plus gown and gloves

Solution or spray for cleaning the skin

Local anaesthetic, syringe and needle

A dressing and strapping — the sterile film type of dressing is ideal

A vial of heparin and ampoule or infusion pack of sterile normal saline

A selection of cannulae — these may be specifically designed arterial cannulae, or suitable intravenous types of sizes no greater than 19G because of the danger of arterial occlusion and subsequent peripheral tissue damage and loss of function.

A flushing device may be used to keep the line patent. These are pre-packed, single-use items.

A single-use 'dome' incorporating a pressure-sensitive membrane, which is linked to the pressure transducer

The pressure transducer monitor. The monitor may need to be checked and calibrated before use.

Commonly used sites for arterial cannulation are the radial and dorsalis pedis arteries. Because of the risk of arterial occlusion, collateral circulation must be tested. The anaesthetist will locate the artery and apply firm pressure until blanching occurs. Normal coloration should return within seconds of releasing the pressure if collateral arterial circulation is adequate.

*Procedure*

The skin is cleaned and anaesthetized in the usual way. The cannula is inserted, and again, the entry site may be sprayed with an antibiotic or iodine preparation before a sterile dressing is applied. The arterial cannula must be clearly identified; it must NEVER be used for intravenous injections because of the danger of sclerosis in the arterioles and capillaries. For this reason some anaesthetists will not use a cannula with an injection port, and some may like to mark the arterial cannula with, for example, red tape.

Once the cannula is in position, it may be attached to the dome, transducer, and monitor, with the flushing device incorporated. The monitor will then give a continual oscilloscope or digital display of arterial pressure.

Complications

*Arterial occlusion.* Either as a result of the use of too large a cannula, or of damage to the vessel wall. Tissue necrosis distally, and loss of function of the hand or foot may result.

*Infection.*

*Inadvertent injection of drugs.*

## CARE OF THE PATIENT ON A VENTILATOR

If a patient needs to receive artificial ventilation for longer than the period of general anaesthesia for surgery, she will usually be transferred to an intensive care unit. However, she will need care during the interim period. A PVC endotracheal tube will normally be used, since this causes less irritation than a rubber tube. If ventilation is likely to be required for a period of days rather than hours, a tracheostomy may be performed, though newer types of endotracheal tube which cause less local irritation or tissue damage may often remain in position for over a week.

The obstetric patient needing an extended period of artificial ventilation may be the eclamptic patient, where maintenance of light anaesthesia will help prevent further fits until cerebral oedema can be reduced and the eclampsia controlled. Following anaesthetic problems, such as inhalation of regurgitated stomach contents or failed intubation with hypoxia, it may be appropriate to ventilate the patient.

The artificially ventilated patient clearly requires the basic nursing care given to any unconscious patient, with particular attention to positioning of the limbs, care of pressure areas, and eye and mouth care. The patient will either be ventilated with anaesthetic gases to keep her lightly anaesthetized, if this is only required for a short period, or she may be given sedatives and perhaps also a muscle relaxant to prevent reflex objection to the endotracheal tube. Restlessness, coughing and attempts to breathe, shown by interruption of the ventilator rhythm, should be reported promptly to the anaesthetist.

Tracheal suction is performed if necessary using aseptic technique. A supply of single sterile disposable gloves and fine suction catheters, also sterile, is required, plus a disposal bag. The nurse washes her hands, explains the procedure to the patient, even if she appears to be unconscious, attaches a clean catheter to the suction apparatus and turns the suction on; she puts a sterile glove on her right hand if she is right-handed. Taking the catheter from its packet and pinching it, she gently inserts it, either via the suction port on the endotracheal tube connector or by carefully detaching the endotracheal or tracheostomy tube from the circuit tubing at this point. Pinching the catheter as it is inserted is essential to prevent trauma to the mucosa. She feeds the catheter down the trachea and then releases the pinching grip so that suction may be performed as she withdraws the catheter. As she removes the used catheter, she coils it up in her hand, then peels off her glove, encasing the soiled catheter, and disposes of both. She now replaces the cap on the suction port, or reconnects the endotracheal tube. The tube should be firmly taped in position, and care must be taken not to displace it at all.

The patient's lungs may be inflated with air, an air/oxygen mixture or added anaesthetic gases. These gases will need to be humidified, and a humidifier will be included in the ventilator circuit. After a period of time, water will collect in the ventilator tubing. For this reason a loop of ventilator tubing should be below the level of the patient's chest. Tubing is disconnected and 'milked' to empty it from time to time. A fluid trap may also be used to catch this excess fluid, and this must be emptied whenever necessary.

Positive End Expiratory Pressure, or PEEP, was mentioned briefly in Chapter 2. It is in the intensive care situation that it is likely to be used, rather than in routine obstetric anaesthesia. PEEP is a means of keeping airway pressure above atmospheric pressure at the end of the expiratory phase, thus opening up collapsed alveoli and improving oxygenation. It may be used for patients with pulmonary oedema, for example, in Mendelson's syndrome, or for any situation where, despite oxygen concentrations of up to 50%, the $PO_2$ remains low or falls. Oxygen concentrations of over 50% are not usually used, since this may lead to oxygen toxicity. Many midwives will be familiar with PEEP as used in neonatal intensive care for babies with respiratory distress syndrome; the principle is the same.

It must be remembered that the artificially ventilated patient may appear unconscious, but may be aware. This must be explained to relatives, who will need much support and reassurance in this situation. The array of equipment around them will seem less horrific if its use is explained, and they should be encouraged to hold the patient's hand and to talk to her. Given prompt and appropriate treatment, newly delivered women do seem, as a rule, to have a great propensity for recovering rapidly from an acute crisis, and optimism is usually justified, though hopes must not be raised unrealistically.

82     *Nursing Responsibilities*

## SUGGESTED FURTHER READING

Campbell, D. and Spence, A. A. (1978) *Anaesthesia, Resuscitation and Intensive Care*. Edinburgh: Churchill Livingstone.

Clarke, D. B. and Barnes, A. D. (1980) *Intensive Care for Nurses*. Oxford: Blackwell Scientific Publications.

Dixon, E. (1983) *Theatre Technique* (Nurses' Aids Series) 5th edn. London: Baillière Tindall.

Kratz, C. (1979) *The Nursing Process*, 1st edn. London: Baillière Tindall.

Sellick, R. A. (1961) Cricoid pressure to control regurgitation of stomach contents during induction of anaesthesia: preliminary communication. *Lancet* ii:404.

Stoddart, J. C. (1975) *Intensive Therapy*. Oxford: Blackwell Scientific Publications.

Tunstall, M. E. (1976) Failed intubation drill. *Anaesthesia* 31:850.

Wachstein, J. and Smith, J. A. H. (1981) *Anaesthesia and Recovery Room Techniques* (Nurses' Aids Series), 3rd edn. London: Baillière Tindall.

Wallace, C. J. (1981) *Anaesthetic Nursing*, 1st edn. London: Pitman Medical.

# 8 Problems in Obstetric Anaesthesia

It may seem strange that obstetric patients, usually young, fit, healthy women, at least in the western world, should present the anaesthetist with any problems, particularly when compared with the patients he will meet in the course of a general surgical list. However, most problems encountered in obstetric anaesthesia arise as the result of the physiological or mechanical effects of pregnancy. They often occur in the patient who presents in an emergency situation or who has had no ante-natal care. These problems will be considered under the following headings:

Acid aspiration or Mendelson's syndrome
Aortocaval occlusion
Difficult intubation
Blood loss

## ACID ASPIRATION OR MENDELSON'S SYNDROME

Silent regurgitation of stomach contents readily occurs during anaesthesia performed on a pregnant woman at term. If these acid stomach contents are inhaled a chemical pneumonitis occurs; this causes bronchospasm, with cyanosis, hypotension, pulmonary oedema and, finally, cardiac failure. The action of proteolytic enzymes in the gastric juice on alveolar tissue is often irreversible, causing reduced efficiency of gaseous exchange.

### Causes

*Reduced Gastric Motility and Delayed Gastric Emptying in Labour*
Although the patient may have taken only fluids during labour, or have been completely starved prior to an elective procedure, some stomach contents will usually be present, and the stomach may be full. Because of the delayed emptying of the stomach, caused by the effect of progesterone and increased by the use of narcotic analgesia,

these contents will be very acid.

## *Laxity of the Oesophageal Sphincter*
Laxity of the oesophageal sphincter also occurs as a result of the effect of progesterone on plain muscle during pregnancy. Pressure from the gravid uterus, particularly with the patient recumbent, may easily cause regurgitation through the relatively lax sphincter. A functional hiatus hernia is often seen in late pregnancy as a result of this pressure, and this increases acid reflux.

## **Prevention**

### *Neutralization of Stomach Contents*
It has been shown that Mendelson's syndrome is unlikely to occur if the pH of gastric contents is above 2.5. It is currently common practice to give routine antacid therapy to all patients in labour in order to achieve and maintain this higher pH. It is also usual, of course, to give patients in established labour fluids only. In some centres mist. magnesium trisilicate 15 ml is given every two hours. Sodium citrate 0.3 molar is thought by some to be more effective, and 30 ml may be given in a similar regime, or alternatively two doses may be given prior to general anaesthesia. Alkaline stomach contents may play some part in improving gastro-oesophageal tone. However, should alkaline stomach contents be regurgitated and aspirated, a similar pathology may ensue, and the particles in mist. magnesium trisilicate, if this is used, may irritate the lungs.

Some recommend turning the patient from side to side to ensure mixing of stomach contents and therefore uniform neutralization.

Cimetidine or ranitidine may be given to inhibit secretion of gastric hydrocholoric acid. A secondary effect of these drugs is a reduction of gastric contents by improving muscle tone and therefore gastric motility. Neither drug neutralizes the stomach contents already present.

### *Emptying of the Stomach*
Because stomach contents will be found in every patient in labour, even if she has been starved, some anaesthetists advocate the use of a Ryles tube pre-operatively, in order to empty the stomach. A wide-bore nasogastric tube is used, and a dose of antacid may be instilled once aspiration has been completed. Some feel, however, that as well as being distressing for the patient, the use of a nasogastric tube may

increase the risk of gastro-oesophageal reflux, and they may reserve this measure for the patient whose recently eaten meal must be removed. Metoclopramide improves gastric motility and aids gastric emptying.

*Protection of the Airway from Gastric Contents*
There are two approaches to this:

*i) Efficient use of cricoid pressure.* Cricoid pressure utilizes the cricoid cartilage, a complete ring of cartilage, to compress the oesophagus against the cervical spine and so prevent regurgitation during induction of anaesthesia. Cricoid pressure is maintained until an endotracheal tube has been passed and its cuff inflated to provide an efficient seal in the trachea (see Chapter 7).

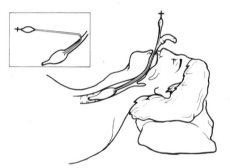

**Fig. 8.1** An endotracheal tube in position. This diagram shows a cuffed, oral endotracheal tube in position, with its cuff inflated, so protecting the airway from regurgitated stomach contents.

*ii) Use of a cuffed endotracheal tube.* The inflated cuff of the endotracheal tube fills the lumen of the trachea, so preventing aspiration even if regurgitation should occur (Fig. 8.1).

**Treatment**
Aspiration of a very small quantity of gastric contents is sufficient to cause the irritant pneumonitis already described, and regurgitation and

aspiration may occur unnoticed. Signs and symptoms usually arise within a short period of time; the patient will become cyanosed, hypotensive and dyspnoeic, and will have a tachycardia. Pulmonary oedema and bronchospasm occur. The arterial $PO_2$ falls, and metabolic acidosis results. A chest X-ray shows pulmonary oedema and atelectasis. In severe cases treatment is ineffective because of the extensive damage to the alveoli.

*Steroid therapy.* This may be effective in reducing alveolar inflammation.
*Artificial ventilation.* The patient is likely to be transferred to an intensive therapy unit where all monitoring and investigations can be carried out easily. Artificial ventilation of the lungs will be needed until the patient can be 'weaned off' the ventilator without an undue fall in arterial $PO_2$. Inflation of the lungs is often a problem and a higher pressure than normal may be required; positive end expiratory pressure (PEEP) may also be necessary (see Chapter 7).
*Palliative measures.* Bronchodilators may be used; antibiotics may be prescribed. Diuretics and digoxin will be necessary if cardiac failure occurs. Intravenous therapy will obviously be required.
*Investigations.* Serial arterial blood gas estimations and regular chest X-rays will give an indication of progress.

## AORTOCAVAL OCCLUSION

### Cause
Aortocaval occlusion may be referred to as 'supine hypotensive syndrome', but this is a misnomer, since occlusion with reduced cardiac output and placental blood flow may occur without a fall in maternal blood pressure. When the pregnant woman in the third trimester lies supine, the weight of the gravid uterus on the major vessels will cause a degree of occlusion, firstly to the vena cava and secondly to the aorta. Reduction of blood flow in the vena cava causes a drop in venous return, reduced cardiac output and often hypotension. Collateral circulation may compensate for this for a short time, but such compensation is not normally well maintained. While the compensatory mechanism is functioning, aortocaval occlusion is said to be concealed, and the patient is normotensive, but when the patient exhibits signs and symptoms, it is 'revealed'. In this case the patient is pale and sweaty and complains of nausea and dizziness. Placental blood flow tends to be compromised early in this situation, and any fetal distress already present

is exacerbated. Aortocaval occlusion combined with any other source of stress, such as maternal hypoxia in difficult intubation, fetal hypoxia in placental insufficiency or hypertonic uterine activity, may well cause maternal or fetal morbidity or mortality. Maternal hypoxia and hypotension occurring simultaneously may lead to cardiac arrest. Hypotension to a greater or lesser degree may be seen following epidural or spinal anaesthesia, and care must be taken that this is not compounded by aortocaval occlusion.

### Prevention

No woman in the third trimester of pregnancy should lie supine for more than a few moments. Fortunately patients usually find it uncomfortable to do so. A wedge may be placed under the mattress on the labour ward bed, or a rolled towel may be placed under the buttocks. Care must be taken to ensure that the wedge actually tilts the patient, so that the uterus is displaced laterally. Patients are frequently happier in a lateral or sitting position in labour, if not actually ambulant. In the operating theatre the table will tilt laterally, and the patient should be transported, whenever this is necessary, lying on her side. The lithotomy position may be a cause of aortocaval occlusion, and again a wedge should be used to tilt the patient.

### Treatment

If the patient suddenly becomes pale, sweaty, nauseated and dizzy, she should be turned onto her side, oxygen should be given by face mask, and the intravenous infusion, if present, may be run more rapidly for a time. The obstetrician should be informed, and also the anaesthetist, if the episode relates to an epidural top-up or any other anaesthetic incident. Maternal blood pressure and fetal heart rate are carefully monitored following such an event, and care is taken to prevent recurrence.

### DIFFICULT INTUBATION

Difficulty in passing an endotracheal tube may be anticipated or unexpected. Any history of surgery or trauma to jaw or neck may lead the anaesthetist to anticipate some anatomical distortion or limitation of movement of the jaw or neck. Part of the anaesthetist's history-taking is therefore likely to include his asking the patient to demonstrate her ability to open her mouth widely! Occasionally congenital abnormalities or physical disabilities, which lead to reduced mobility of the cervical

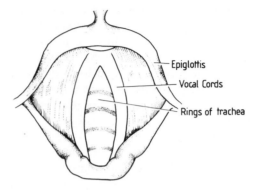

**Fig. 8.2** The larynx and vocal cords as seen at laryngoscopy.

spine, may be seen, and micrognathia is also likely to cause difficulty. Such problems may cause difficulty in visualizing the cords on laryngoscopy (Fig. 8.2); intubation then has to be performed 'blind'. Evidence of surgery on the neck may easily be missed, since neck scars heal well and are usually managed post-operatively so as to give good cosmetic results. Unless the patient is questioned carefully, she may fail to see the relevance of such surgery to her pregnancy and may not think it worthy of mention at ante-natal booking, particularly if the surgery was performed some years earlier.

The other group of patients who may be difficult to intubate are those suffering from pre-eclampsia or eclampsia, and demonstrating anything more than a moderate degree of oedema. These women are likely to have laryngeal oedema; unfortunately they are also very likely to require general anaesthesia for caesarean section.

The obese patient is never the ideal candidate for general anaesthesia, but the short, stocky or overweight woman more often than not seems unable to deliver spontaneously. For purely physical and mechanical reasons, the cords may again be difficult to visualize in the patient with a short, 'thick' neck.

Because difficulty with intubation can occur when least expected, it is generally recommended that all patients be pre-oxygenated before induction of general anaesthesia for caesarean section. Pregnant women become hypoxic more rapidly during a period of apnoea than non-pregnant women. The fetus is likely to suffer hypoxia before the mother does, and if caesarean section is being performed because of fetal distress, this will be exacerbated. Pre-oxygenation is continued for a full three minutes at the very least, and five minutes is frequently advocated. Oxygen is given via a non-rebreathing circuit, such as the Magill circuit, at a rate of 8 litres per minute. Pre-oxygenation should be uninterrupted and it should be timed. The patient may hold the mask on for herself if she prefers this, and she should be encouraged to hold it firmly in place so that air does not enter around the mask. Many patients will dislike the face mask because they feel claustrophobic and generally distressed. The patient may feel extremely uncomfortable lying flat (apart from the lateral tilt of the table) and efforts must be made to minimize her distress, perhaps by raising her head, by the use of a lighter, clear face mask, such as the Ambu mask, and certainly by giving her support and reassurance.

Although pre-oxygenation performed as a routine measure should reduce the incidence of severe hypoxia this is by no means the end of the matter. Failure to intubate the trachea occurs when the patient has received an intravenous anaesthetic agent and a muscle relaxant, usually a short-acting agent such as suxamethonium. She is therefore paralysed and cannot be oxygenated while attempts at intubation continue. Repeated attempts to intubate may lead to local trauma, thus compounding the problem. A degree of hypoxia is inevitable over a period of time, and regurgitation may occur to complicate matters.

If the anaesthetist is able to obtain a good airway and ventilate the lungs adequately using an airway and face mask, he may ask his assistant to maintain cricoid pressure, and continue the anaesthetic by this means. He will ventilate the patient's lungs manually until the effects of the muscle relaxant have worn off, after which the patient will breathe spontaneously. He may wish to pass a nasogastric tube and empty the stomach in this situation.

If a good airway is not easily maintained, the anaesthetist will usually elect to allow the patient to wake up. If the caesarean section is not urgent, it may be deferred; if surgery must proceed, it will usually be performed under spinal anaesthesia. Spinal anaesthesia is the preferred alternative, partly because of its rapidity of onset and relative ease of performance, but also because an accidental 'total spinal' block occurring during an attempted epidural block would, in turn, necessitate endotracheal intubation.

Every situation has to be assessed as it arises. The decision may be a very difficult one, but although it is understandably an emotive subject, it is usual to consider the mother's well-being before that of her baby in this complex situation.

Some centres carry 'difficult intubation' equipment, with a selection of sizes and types of endotracheal tubes, laryngoscopes and introducers, plus equipment for performing tracheostomy. Some anaesthetists feel that the provision of such facilities may lead the less experienced anaesthetist to persevere for too long with attempts to intubate the patient. This has been pinpointed as the cause of death in some instances, as a result of the severe hypoxia caused.

However, the range of different endotracheal tubes and laryngoscopes may allow the anaesthetist to select the appropriate equipment for any given difficulty he is experiencing. Various patterns of laryngoscope may enable him to visualize the cords if this is a problem. Introducers may be of wire, with a guard to prevent protrusion and damage to the trachea, and these allow the endotracheal tube to be 'moulded' slightly to facilitate direction of the tip. Introducers of such materials as rubber, gum elastic or silastic may be used protruding from the end of the endotracheal tube, so that the tip of the introducer can 'lead' the tube through the cords, and the tube is then passed down over it.

## BLOOD LOSS

Haemorrhage in obstetrics may be sudden and severe, whether it occurs before or after delivery. The patient may frequently require urgent surgery but may not be fit for immediate anaesthesia. She may have had no ante-natal care, or she may be away from home so that no full medical notes are available. She may be profoundly shocked or distressed, and if she is unaccompanied by a close relative, no adequate medical and obstetric history may be obtainable. Blood loss over a period of time is usually partially compensated for and is therefore less devastating, but massive haemorrhage occurring in a short space of time can have long-term effects on other systems, notably renal function. Renal failure may become a chronic problem, and pituitary failure (Sheehan's syndrome) may also occur.

Having said this, the physiological changes in pregnancy and, indeed, at delivery do compensate for blood loss to a certain extent, so that the pregnant patient seems better able to withstand and recover from haemorrhage than her non-pregnant counterpart. These physiological changes are complex and closely interrelated, and changes in any one system therefore cannot be looked at in isolation. However, the increased circulating volume is a relevant factor in the consideration of blood loss. Plasma volume increases by 50% in a full term pregnancy, while red cell volume increases by considerably less — 18% — resulting in a degree of haemodilution. The increase in red cells is thought to be partly dependent on iron and folic acid supplements. Despite a reduction in haematocrit and red cell volume, the platelet count probably remains at about the pre-pregnancy level. Clotting occurs more readily, probably in preparation for the third stage of labour, but the complications arising from this include the increased risk of deep vein thrombosis and also of disseminated intravascular coagulation (DIC) once haemorrhage has occurred.

Occasionally a patient is found to have a sub-clinical coagulation defect, asymptomatic until delivery. Alongside the hypercoagulability of the blood in pregnancy the problem of hypofibrinogenaemia must be considered. When an intensive coagulation situation arises, such as formation of a retroplacental clot in placental abruption, fibrinogen levels fall, so that fibrin will not be produced. Clotting will not occur, and bleeding will result. Coagulation mechanisms and fibrinolysis usually co-exist in equilibrium to prevent coagulation within the system, and the fibrinolysis described above will tend to limit DIC, although leading to excessive blood loss at delivery. Once diagnosed hypofibrinogenaemia is treated by transfusion of fibrinogen in solution.

The physiological reaction to blood loss is peripheral vasoconstriction; this eventually leads to tissue hypoxia, and metabolic acidosis results. It is this acidosis which causes damage to and malfunction of vital systems, and cardiac arrhythmias or even cardiac arrest may occur. This is the extreme stage of shock, and is known as intractable or irreversible shock.

**Fluid Replacement Therapy**

Fluid replacement therapy following haemorrhage has to be both quantitative and qualitative.

Accurate replacement of circulating volume is monitored by observation of central venous pressure. Overloading the circulation places strain on the cardiopulmonary system and must be avoided.

Accurate replacement of circulating contents is aided by assessment of actual blood loss and frequent reassessment of haematological values and electrolytes. There are various problems associated with the giving of large amounts of stored blood from the blood bank. Incompatibility is not as big a problem as in the past thanks to sophisticated cross-matching techniques, though all checking procedures must be carried out meticulously and the patient observed carefully during transfusion. Even so, 'hypertransfusion syndrome' may occur. In this instance, because platelets and certain clotting factors are not viable in storage conditions, the patient's blood volume may be restored, but with blood deficient in clotting factors, thus giving her an overall coagulation defect. She will therefore tend to continue bleeding, and the problem is compounded. This is prevented by supplementing cross-matched blood with fresh-frozen plasma and platelets when necessary. Once detailed clotting studies can be performed, some deficiencies of specific clotting factors may be remedied by transfusion of the appropriate factor in solution. For these reasons, although blood will certainly be cross-matched in appropriate quantities, blood loss will initially be treated by the use of plasma expanders (or substitutes) and blood derivatives. Clear fluids are useful for the immediate treatment of shock. However, they remain in the circulation for a limited period, and so may be used in conjunction with other types of intravenous fluids. Intravenous fluids commonly used include:

*Blood and Blood Derivatives*

*Cross-matched 'bank' blood — 'hyper-transfusion syndrome' and incompatibility or allergic reactions.* These have already been mentioned. All bank blood is now tested for serum hepatitis as a routine, so this risk is very much reduced.

Rapid transfusion may cause a raised serum potassium level, which will be significant if renal function is impaired. The citrate compound used as an anti-coagulant in bank blood may cause a metabolic alkalosis, and this results in a temporary reduction in the oxygen transport efficiency of the red cells. Micro-emboli may be a problem and blood filters should be used whenever blood is transfused.

*Packed cells.* In general this form of blood carries the same risks as whole blood. Packed cells are often given to the anaemic patient who does not require extra volume, but whose oxygen transport efficiency is reduced.

*Fresh frozen plasma (FFP).* Most coagulation factors are present, but FFP contains no platelets.

*Human Plasma Protein Fraction (HPPF).* This is pasteurized during preparation, and so serum hepatitis should not be a risk. Micro-emboli are not present. HPPF can be stored safely for up to two years. It remains in the circulation for about 24 hours, so maintaining circulatory volume.

*Salt-poor albumin.* This is expensive and not readily available, but is useful for patients with cardiac or renal impairment.

*Platelets.* Once a certain quantity of stored blood has been transfused, platelets may also be given. Platelet transfusion is expensive, and this facility may not be readily available.

*Fibrinogen.* This is available for patients with known hypofibrinogenaemia.

*Specific clotting factors.* Many of these have been isolated and can be transfused to correct known deficiencies.

*Plasma Expanders or Plasma Substitutes*

*The dextrans.* The dextrans are available in low, medium and high molecular weights in the UK — Dextran 40, Dextran 70 and Dextran 110, respectively. Each of these is available in normal saline or 5% dextrose.

Dextran 40 remains in circulation for only about 3–4 hours and is excreted in the urine. Dextran 70 and Dextran 110 are metabolized to glucose after a longer period, and maintain circulatory volume for 12–36 hours.

Although dextrans are very useful as 'plasma expanders', excessive use of these substances will cause haemodilution, leading to reduced oxygen-carrying efficiency, and this necessitates increased cardiac output to meet oxygen requirements. For this reason it is usual to give a maximum of one litre of dextran. Dextrans of high molecular weight may interfere with subsequent cross-matching of blood; they may cause coagulation defects and occasionally give rise to an anaphylactic reaction.

*Haemaccel.* This boosts circulating volume for a shorter period and so is useful in early treatment. It is excreted after 1–4 hours. Anaphylactic reaction may occasionally be a problem.

*Clear fluids.* These remain in circulation for a very short time and diffuse into the tissues or are excreted after only 20–30 minutes. However, they are necessary for replacement of electrolytes and calories. Excessive infusion of clear fluids may cause 'water intoxication' and renal overload.

### Reversal of Metabolic Acidosis

Metabolic acidosis is seen only after major blood loss. Tissue hypoxia results in an anaerobic form of metabolism within the cells, the end products of which are various acids, such as lactic acid. Once this has occurred, treatment may need to be given to restore the pH of the blood to 7.4, in which case sodium bicarbonate 8.4% is infused intravenously. Prompt restoration of circulating volume with adequate oxygen transport substances will usually obviate the necessity for this extreme treatment. The citrate used in bank blood is metabolized to sodium bicarbonate by the body, causing alkalosis. Dextrose and insulin therapy may be necessary to restore general metabolic balance.

### Peripheral Vasodilatation

After severe haemorrhage the normal physiological response of peripheral vasoconstriction, a physiological economy designed to protect vital organs and prevent central hypoxia, may be slow to reverse despite restoration of circulatory volume. Failure to reverse this reaction will result in central circulatory overload with cardiopulmonary embarrassment, and continued metabolic acidosis. Steroids may be useful, and are given in high doses.

### SUGGESTED FURTHER READING

Crawford, J. S. (1970) The anaesthetist's contribution to maternal mortality. *British Journal of Anaesthesia* 42:70.

Crawford, J. S. (1978) *Principles and Practice of Obstetric Anaesthesia,* 4th edn. Oxford: Blackwell Scientific Publications.

Department of Health and Social Security. *Report on Confidential Enquiries into Maternal Deaths in England and Wales (1973–75).* London: HMSO.

Department of Health and Social Security. *Report on Confidential Enquiries into Maternal Deaths in England and Wales (1976–78).* London: HMSO.

Husemeyer, R. P., Davenport, H. T. and Rajasekaren, T. (1978) Cimetidine as a single oral dose for prophylaxis against Mendelson's syndrome. *Anaesthesia* 33:775.

Lahiri, S. K., Thomas, T. A. and Hodgson, R. M. H. (1973) Single-dose antacid therapy for the prevention of Mendelson's syndrome. *British Journal of Anaesthesia* 34:306.

Mackenzie, A. I. (1978) Laryngeal oedema complicating obstetric anaesthesia *Anaesthesia* 33:271.

Moir, D. D. (1980) *Obstetric Anaesthesia and Analgesia,* 2nd edn. London: Baillière Tindall.

Sellick, R. A. (1961) Cricoid pressure to control regurgitation of stomach contents during induction of anaesthesia: preliminary communication. *Lancet* ii:404.

Tunstall, M. E. (1976) Failed intubation drill. *Anaesthesia* 31:850.

Turndorf, H., Rodis, I. D., and Clark, T. S. (1974) 'Silent' regurgitation during general anaesthesia. *Anaesthesia and Analgesia, Current Research* 53:700.

# 9 *Obstetric Analgesia*

Pain is a subjective experience; it is different things to different people, and it is therefore impossible to qualify. The only person who may reasonably define pain is the one experiencing it. Pain is assessed by the effect it is having on the sufferer, since this determines the kind of treatment necessary. The degree to which any type of pain affects its victim is modified by that person's temperament, mental state, environment and background, as well as by other physical factors. Fear and anxiety will tend to exacerbate pain; various forms of distraction can play a part in alleviating it.

In the context of day-to-day living, pain has a protective function. Thus the reception and transmission of painful stimuli will result in a part of the body being removed instantly from a source of injury, such as a hot saucepan handle. Infection, for example, will lead to inflammation, which causes pain and therefore limits movement, so that the affected part will be rested, allowing the body's defence mechanisms to function more efficiently and to localize and fight the infection.

## Pain Pathways

The sensory nerve endings in the skin normally transmit clearly defined pain sensations, so that both the type and location of pain can be accurately described. Similar pain receptors are found in the peritoneum and in the outer layers of the abdominal and pelvic organs. However, these deeper structures do not have nerve endings within them, and pain arising from inflammation or pressure within any abdominal organ tends to be ill defined and is often referred. For example, pain arising from the gall bladder may be referred to the shoulder. Such pain, originating in the abdominal or pelvic organs, is known as visceral pain.

The ascending sensory tract is described in three stages (Fig. 9.1). The first neurone is located in the posterior or dorsal root ganglion of one of the spinal nerves. Its dendron goes to the skin to form the receptor, while its axon goes to the posterior horn of the spinal cord.

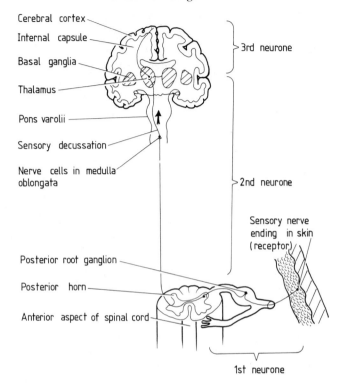

Cerebral cortex
Internal capsule
Basal ganglia
Thalamus
Pons varolii
Sensory decussation
Nerve cells in medulla oblongata
3rd neurone
2nd neurone
Sensory nerve ending in skin (receptor)
Posterior root ganglion
Posterior horn
Anterior aspect of spinal cord
1st neurone

**Fig. 9.1** The sensory pathway, showing the structures involved in the appreciation of pain.

The second neurone arises in the posterior horn, crosses over within the spinal cord, forming the sensory decussation, and ascends through the medulla, pons and mid-brain to the thalamus. The third neurone arises in the thalamus and transmits the sensory impulse to the sensory cortex, where the impulse is translated.

Nerves may be myelinated or non-myelinated. The myelin sheath is the outer covering of the nerve fibre. In myelinated nerves, it is interrupted at intervals along its length and the gaps so formed are called the nodes of Ranvier. The electrical impulses of nervous activity pass rapidly from one node to the next. This is known as saltatory conduction, and transmission of impulses in this way is much more rapid than that occurring along non-myelinated nerves. Larger, myelinated nerves are often known as 'A' fibres; these transmit acute or sharp pain sensation along the sensory pathway already described, to the sensory area of the cerebral cortex. The slower, slightly smaller, unmyelinated 'C' fibres carry duller, less acute pain sensation, and these sensations travel to the cortex by a more circuitous route. Sensation travelling along 'C' fibres is more liable to be interrupted or modified by other impulses. This is known as the 'gate control' theory.

*Gate Control Theory*
The gate control theory suggests that sensory impulses 'open' the gate, i.e. allow transmission of impulses up the sensory tract in the spinal cord. The passage of other impulses along larger nerve fibres may supersede the original impulse and close the gate, thus preventing transmission to the cortex. This is the theory underlying the use of a transcutaneous nerve stimulator in intractable pain, where a variable electrical stimulus is applied over the nerves transmitting the pain sensation. Another example is the use of a cold spray for sports injuries. The reception and transmission of the sensation of extreme cold blocks the transmission of the pain sensation. It is thought that 'gate control' also operates higher in the sensory tract, i.e. in the mid-brain and thalamus. Before 'gate control' is activated, sensation is assessed in the cortex and qualified in the light of past experience and present expectation, with anxiety, fear and cultural factors also playing a part.

*Prostaglandins*
Pain receptors are stimulated not only by direct trauma but also by various substances released by inflamed tissue. One such substance is a member of the prostaglandin group.

*Endogenous Opiates*
An exciting discovery in recent years has been that of opiate receptors in the central nervous system. These are cells to which opiates attach themselves to produce their effect. Such receptors are found along the 'pain pathways', in the spinal cord, thalamus and mid-brain; they are also found in the respiratory centre in the thalamus, hence the respiratory depressant effect of the opiate drugs. The endogenous opiates which combine with these receptors under the stress of trauma or pain are secreted in the brain. Two main types are described:
i) Endorphins are found mainly in the hypothalamus and the pituitary gland.

ii) Enkephalins are smaller molecules widely distributed throughout the substance of the brain.

Multiple or severe injuries apparently cause the release of endorphins as well as ACTH from the pituitary gland, and this is thought to be the reason why accident victims are often relatively free of pain or shock.

**Pain Pathways in Labour**
The woman in labour commonly describes her pain as being 'like a bad period pain'. She is often surprised to feel the pain sensation in her lower abdomen and often also in her lower back. The pain may radiate into her groins. At the same time she may be aware of the tightening of her uterus as the contractions occur. The pain of contractions is a result of the unique muscular activity of the myometrium. Contraction of the myometrium causes increased cellular metabolism as energy is required; this results in transient ischaemia causing a cramp-like pain. The uterine nerve supply is linked, via the paracervical plexus, to spinal nerves T11 and T12, the last two thoracic nerves. As uterine contractions radiate down over the uterus from the fundus, in co-ordinate uterine action, so the cervix begins to dilate.

Cervical pain is related to spinal nerves T11 and T12, and as first-stage pain becomes more intense, T10 and L1 are also involved. As labour progresses and the presenting part descends, causing pressure and new sensations of discomfort, pain from the vagina, rectum and perineum will be relayed along the pudendal nerve to the second, third and fourth sacral nerves (S2, S3, S4). The remaining lumbar and sacral nerves will relay pain sensation resulting from pressure throughout the lower abdomen and pelvis, but T10, T11, T12, L1, S2, S3 and S4 are the nerves concerned with pain arising from the birth canal itself (Fig. 9.2).

Just as every labour is different, so the perception of pain varies for every individual woman. Factors affecting this variation include:

Length, strength and frequency of contractions, and duration of labour.
Efficiency of contractions — inco-ordinate uterine action often causes very painful contractions early in labour when the cervix has dilated very little.
Presentation and position of the fetus.
Parity of the woman.
Levels of fear and tension; often attributable to too little or too much knowledge!

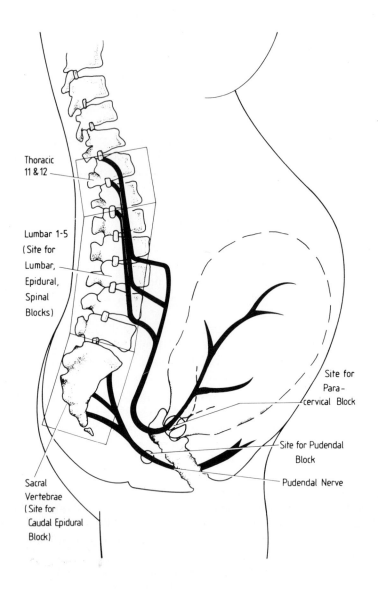

Thoracic 11 & 12

Lumbar 1-5 (Site for Lumbar, Epidural, Spinal Blocks)

Sacral Vertebrae (Site for Caudal Epidural Block)

Site for Para-cervical Block

Site for Pudendal Block

Pudendal Nerve

**Fig. 9.2** Pain pathways in labour, showing the sites at which pain may be intercepted by local anaesthetic techniques.

**Relief of Pain in Labour**

For the woman in labour perhaps the most important factor is the presence of a supportive companion. Happily, these days, for the majority of women this can be the father of her baby, as well as the midwife. Perhaps the most commonly voiced fears apart from the obvious apprehension of the unknown, are "Will I be left alone?" and "Will I be able to cope with the pain?" (often voiced as "Will I make a fool of myself?").

The importance of realistic and pertinent ante-natal preparation for labour and childbirth cannot be overstressed. Rather than glossing over the fact that unaided labour can be a long, painful, distressing ordeal, ante-natal classes need to present the available options in a clear, balanced way. Each analgesic method has its advantages and drawbacks, and those giving ante-natal talks will see the need to present information in an objective way, as far as possible uncoloured by personal feelings.

Every pregnant woman has the right to be assured of treatment to suit her individual requirements in labour and at delivery. The pain relief suited to one woman will be totally unacceptable to another, and if every woman could embark on her labour assured of either the support and encouragement in her chosen method of analgesia, or the guidance she requires towards the right method for her, much stress could be alleviated.

Those involved in giving ante-natal talks will readily recognize the problem of talking to a group. Some women wish to know every fine detail because they fear the unknown, while others wish to put themselves entirely in the hands of the professionals, and to be spared any decision-making. Happily, the work of the National Childbirth Trust (NCT) is well established in the UK now, and this organization does much to inform those who wish to be fully informed and to provide opportunity for debate and discussion, offering a supportive network, both ante-natally and post-natally, as well as giving women and their partners practical help in actively coping with their labours. For those who wish to have less rigorous preparation for labour, midwives and, in an increasing number of centres, physiotherapists provide a less complicated series of relaxation exercises. These are easily taught and recalled, and though details vary, the principles, on the whole, do not. In the foreseeable future, midwives will continue to play an important role in this area of ante-natal preparation, and an understanding of it is vital if support and encouragement are to be given to the woman using her breathing techniques in labour. The Association of Obstetric

Physiotherapists makes a valuable contribution to ante-natal preparation, with a simple, effective curriculum for the expectant mother.

Certainly midwives will not wish to see lay and paramedical groups taking over the area of ante-natal preparation and teaching, and all midwives should feel able to teach relaxation and breathing techniques. Indeed, the ante-natal period is an ideal time for reinforcing more general matters of health education, such as posture and correct lifting techniques, coping with stress, and healthy eating for all the family, to name but a few. The midwife is well equipped to cover this broad base if she combines her professional expertise with common sense.

In recognizing the contribution made by groups such as the NCT and in supporting a woman in her chosen approach to labour (whatever her own feelings may be), the midwife may often find herself dealing with parents who cannot realize their chosen ideals. If a couple have set their sights on 'natural childbirth' with no analgesia, and their ideal proves totally unrealistic, they may need much support in changing course and modifying this ideal. There may be conflict between the couple, as well as an individual sense of guilt and failure.

Breathing and relaxation techniques and exercises, as taught in ante-natal preparation classes throughout the UK and by the NCT and similar groups, have an important part to play in labour. The woman is encouraged to participate actively in her labour rather than lying back and merely enduring the contractions. This active participation acts partly as a distraction therapy, and the resulting relaxation is of course beneficial to both mother and fetus. However, for most primigravidae, the important factors of ante-natal preparation, supportive companionship during labour and effective use of breathing and relaxation techniques will need to be supplemented by more active analgesic methods, and these will now be considered.

The pain caused by uterine contractions in labour and pain at delivery can be treated at various points along the sensory path.

Local infiltration of local anaesthetic solutions interrupts the pain pathway at the point nearest its source, the adjacent receptor or afferent nerve endings. A common example is perineal infiltration.

Regional analgesia tackles the problem at the point where pain is transmitted to the spinal column, and the use of local anaesthetics or opiates in the epidural space or of local anaesthetics in the subarachnoid space will prevent sensation being transmitted beyond the spinal nerves.

The other main analgesic techniques — systemic opiates and inhalational analgesia — have their effect at a cerebral level and inhibit or modify cerebral interpretation and response to painful stimuli.

Hypnotics and tranquillizers are used as adjuncts to analgesics to alleviate tension and to potentiate their effect.

As so-called 'fringe medicine' gains in credibility and popularity, labour may well come to be more commonly conducted under acupuncture. This ancient technique may be linked to the endogenous opiates phenomenon, though it is basically still empirical. Caesarean section has also been performed under acupuncture.

Hypnosis is also used occasionally, and this is a form of distraction therapy.

So-called 'active birth' takes the psychoprophylaxis approach a stage further, encouraging mobility during labour and the assuming of the most comfortable  position for delivery, such as squatting, or leaning forward on all fours. This would seem to be a very valid approach, both psychologically and physiologically, since  it gives the woman freedom of choice, allowing her to feel 'in control' and therefore more able to relax. Physiologically, it makes optimum use of the force of gravity and would seem likely to make the second stage of labour less uncomfortable, if the pressure on the sacrum and coccyx from sitting on a hard bed is removed. The pelvic floor is then likely to be less severely assaulted.

Unfortunately, most Caucasian primigravidae lack the stamina and the self-confidence to benefit from this approach right through labour, though many multiparous women and their babies have undoubtedly done so. 'Active birth' implies active support, and the participation by the partner plays a large part in the success of such an approach, which bears out the theory posed by O'Driscoll and others that the presence of a supportive companion in labour reduces the need for analgesia.

### SUGGESTED FURTHER READING

Atkinson, R. S., Rushman, G. B. and Lee, J. A. (1977) *A Synopsis of Anaesthesia,* 8th edn. Bristol: John Wright.

Bonica, J. J. (1972) *Obstetric Analgesia and Anaesthesia.* Berlin: Springer-Verlag.

Corke, B. C. (1977) Neurobehavioural responses of the newborn: the effect of different forms of maternal analgesia. *Anaesthesia* 32: 539.

Crawford, J. S. (1978) *Principles and Practice of Obstetric Anaesthesia,* 4th edn. Oxford: Blackwell Scientific Publications.

Holdcroft, A. and Morgan, M. (1974) An assessment of the analgesic effect in labour of pethidine and 50% nitrous oxide in oxygen (Entonox). *Journal of Obstetrics and Gynaecology (British Commonwealth)* 81: 603.

Melzack, R. (1973) *The Puzzle of Pain.* Harmondsworth: Penguin Education.

Moir, D. D. (1980) *Obstetric Anaesthesia and Analgesia,* 2nd edn. London: Baillière Tindall.

O'Driscoll, K. (1975) An obstetrician's view on pain. *British Journal of Anaesthesia* 47: 1053.

O'Driscoll, K. and Meagher, D. (1980) *Active Management of Labour* (Supplement to *Clinics in Obstetrics and Gynaecology).* Eastbourne: W. B. Saunders.

Plantevin, O. M. (1973) *Analgesia and Anaesthesia in Obstetrics.* London: Butterworth.

Ross, J. S. and Wilson, K. J. W. (1980) *Foundations in Anatomy and Physiology,* 1st edn. Edinburgh: Churchill Livingstone.

# 10 *Drugs in Labour*

## PARENTERAL NARCOTICS

A narcotic is a drug which produces deadness and induces torpor. The term narcotic is usually reserved for powerful analgesic drugs which act on the central nervous system. Because of their effect on the central nervous system, many of these drugs are addictive, have the potential for abuse, and therefore come under the *Misuse of Drugs Act*. They are the opiate group and their derivatives, natural and synthetic. They are known as opiates because the earliest substances classified in this way, such as morphine, were derived from opium. Narcotics given parenterally (that is, injected) are widely used in labour, but because of the possible side-effects on the fetus, they are reserved for the first stage of labour.

Under the *Misuse of Drugs Regulations 1973* and the *Misuse of Drugs (Amendment) Regulations 1974*, midwives are permitted to use certain controlled drugs at their discretion. These are listed in Schedule iv of the *Medicines (Prescriptions only) Order 1977* and may be supplied to midwives for use in their practice under Part III of the *Medicines Act 1968*. Midwives must adhere to local policy and conform to the rules of the United Kingdom Central Council for Nursing, Midwifery and Health Visiting. These rules are in accordance with those of the former Central Midwives Board and the Northern Ireland Council for Nurses and Midwives. These rules state:

RESTRICTION ON THE USE OF DRUGS

A practising midwife shall not on her own responsibility administer any drug, including an analgesic, unless in the course of her training, whether before or after enrolment, she has been thoroughly instructed in its use, and is familiar with its dosage and methods of administration or application.

DUTY TO RECORD ADMINISTRATION OF DRUGS

A practising midwife who administers or applies in any way any drug other than an aperient, must make a proper record of the name and dose of the drug, and the date, time and method of its administration or application.

FOR NORTHERN IRELAND

A practising midwife shall not, on her own responsibility, administer any controlled medicine, or any inhalational analgesic, unless she has received instruction in its use and the medicine or inhalational analgesic has been approved by the Council as appropriate to the practice of midwifery.

FOR SCOTLAND

A practising midwife shall not administer any controlled drug or medicine unless she is familiar with its dosage, its method of administration and its contra-indications. She shall observe the requirements of current regulations regarding controlled drugs and medicine.

The majority of women in labour in this country, some 70%, depend on narcotic analgesics for pain relief in labour. This is because midwives may use these drugs on their own initiative, and because the technique is simple.

The particular drug used in a hospital is normally the choice of the local obstetricians, and they formulate policies for the use of analgesics in labour. Such policies will stipulate the drugs which may be given and the maximum total doses which may be administered by the midwife. The giving of analgesia beyond such limits becomes a medical decision and requires a doctor's prescription. Generally speaking, equally effective analgesic doses of the majority of currently available drugs are equally depressant to the baby and have a similar profile of side-effects on the mother.

**Pethidine (Meperidine, Demerol).** Although over 40 years old, pethidine is probably still the most widely prescribed analgesic in labour. It does not inhibit uterine contractions in established labour, and there is little foundation for the view that pethidine should not be given early in case labour is inhibited. If uterine contractions cease after administration of pethidine, then labour was not truly established. On the contrary, pethidine probably improves uterine action. It causes nausea and vomiting in up to 50% of cases, and may, on occasion, cause loss of self-control while failing to relieve the pain to any extent, patients may regret its administration for this reason.

It readily crosses the placenta; the fetal /maternal (F/M) ratio approaches and may exceed 1.0 (see Chapter 4). The period of one to three hours after intramuscular injection of pethidine is said to be the time of greatest risk to the baby, while after intravenous injection the drug appears in fetal blood within three minutes.

The intramuscular dose of pethidine is 50–150 mg. There are two schools of thought regarding dosage. In those units where active management of labour is practised, where the mother is assured of delivery within 8 hours of being admitted to the unit in established labour, and where other methods of pain relief are offered if pethidine is unsatisfactory, 50 mg repeated, if necessary, 30 minutes later seems to be effective for many women. Others believe that a large initial dose of 150 mg is likely to be more effective and will gain the mother's confidence. There seems little doubt that sympathetic support from the midwife and the presence of the woman's husband or a relative reduce analgesic requirement.

Whatever dosage regime is used, the effectiveness of pethidine in relieving pain has been questioned. It certainly does not relieve pain as completely as does an epidural. Estimates of 40% of patients failing to receive satisfactory analgesia have been given. Assessment of analgesia is of course very difficult. The woman who has received judicious analgesia in labour has probably also experienced intensification of pain at about the same time and may fail to appreciate this or to take it into account when considering the relief of her pain. Such assessment also depends on whether women assess the pain while actually in labour, or at some time following delivery. Happily, the more painful parts of labour tend to be forgotten with the passage of time.

One problem with the use of pethidine is that standard doses tend to be given to all women. A standard dose, say 100 mg, may be appropriate for an average-sized individual, but inadequate for a larger woman and too much for a small one. For this reason, the use of titrated doses of intravenous pethidine has been advocated on the basis that each patient will thus receive enough pethidine to relieve pain, but not enough to cause side-effects. The problem with this is that it requires medical participation, and it has therefore met with understandable resistance. To overcome this problem, a machine has been developed (the Cardiff Palliator); this delivers set amounts of pethidine from a syringe pump at the mother's request. After insertion of an intravenous line and connection to the device, the patient can give herself 1 ml of solution containing 25 mg of pethidine as long as she pushes the button in a certain way. This prevents her giving herself a dose if she is semi-conscious, and she cannot give herself a dose more frequently than once every ten minutes; there are other inbuilt safeguards to prevent overdose. In a trial using the machine, mothers obtained good analgesia at lower total doses than another group given intramuscular pethidine. However, a significant proportion suffered nausea and vomiting.

**Diamorphine.** Although a powerful opiate which may cause marked depression of the infant, diamorphine causes relaxation and euphoria, and may be useful in labour. It is normally given with caution in the UK because the risk of addiction is feared, but those who favour its use will argue that this risk is minimal after one or two doses given during labour. With the increasing availability of epidural analgesia, it is likely to be used less as time goes on.

**Pentazocine (Fortral).** This is also a drug which may be prescribed by midwives. Like pethidine, it is a strong analgesic. It enhances uterine contractility and also tends to cause nausea and vomiting, at least after one dose, though this is less of a problem after two or more doses. It is very unlikely to cause addiction and does not come under the *Misuse of Drugs Act.* It seems to cross the placenta to a lesser extent than pethidine. Certainly there is less depression of infants of mothers given two or more doses of pentazocine, compared with infants whose mothers received pethidine. Dosage is 40–60 mg, 40 mg being equivalent to 100 mg of pethidine. The injection is irritant. Pentazocine has failed to supplant pethidine because of undesirable side-effects such as hallucinations and sweating.

**Morphine.** This was the classic drug used for prolonged and painful labour, particularly in primigravidae, since it has the advantage over pethidine of relieving anxiety. It does, however, cause greater depression of the respiratory centre of the infant in equi-analgesic doses. With the trend towards shorter labours and the greater use of epidurals, morphine has all but disappeared from the labour wards, though it is still used to give pain relief following concealed ante-partum haemorrhage.

There are two classes of drugs which are often combined with narcotic analgesics in an effort to reduce the incidence of side-effects.

## Narcotic Antagonists

These are drugs which reverse the effects of narcotics. A combination of the two was suggested on the basis that, in theory, there would be maximal analgesia with minimal respiratory depression of both the mother and her infant. The most popular combination is Pethilorfan, a mixture of pethidine 100 mg with levallorphan 1.25 mg in 2 ml, a drug approved for prescription by midwives. Unfortunately, the antagonist does reduce the analgesic potency of the narcotic, and equi-analgesic doses of pethidine and Pethilorfan are equally depressant. There is little if any place for Pethilorfan in modern obstetrics in the UK.

This is not to say there is no place for narcotic antagonists. They are given to the baby known or thought to be depressed by narcotics. In this situation, the antagonist of choice is naloxone (Narcan). It is specific, i.e. it has no action unless there is narcotic present in the baby. It is the only drug which reverses the effects of pentazocine. One intramuscular dose given to the infant of a mother who has received pethidine during labour reverses the adverse effects of the narcotic to the extent that the baby's ability to suck and his neurobehavioural scores will be normal (see Chapter 4). In some units naloxone is given to all babies whose mothers have received pethidine during labour. Naloxone has a fairly short duration of action in adults but a longer one in neonates, so that there is little risk of the effect of the naloxone wearing off before that of the narcotic. Neonatal naloxone is supplied in ampoules containing 0.04 mg per ml, and dosage is usually 0.04 mg (1 ml) for an infant at term.

Other narcotic antagonists are levallorphan and nalorphine, but they may have a respiratory depressant effect themselves if given to a baby who is not depressed by narcotics. Naloxone has now largely replaced these two drugs.

## Tranquillizers.

Tranquillizers may be given with narcotics in labour for three reasons:
i) By potentiating the effects of pethidine, analgesia is obtained with lower doses.
ii) Anxiety is relieved.
iii) The incidence of nausea and vomiting is reduced.

Two popular drugs are promazine (Sparine) and promethazine (Phenergan). These cross the placenta very easily, and their effects persist in the baby for some time, further adding to the depressant effect of the narcotic used. Anxiety in labour is perhaps better treated, in the majority of cases, by sympathetic support and reassurance, while nausea and vomiting should ideally be treated as they arise, using a specific anti-emetic such as prochlorperazine (Stemetil) or perphenazine (Fentazin). The latter drugs must be prescribed by a doctor, whereas midwives may be authorized to give promazine or promethazine to patients in labour.

Diazepam has been used to reduce anxiety in labour, but it was found that total doses in excess of 30 mg to the mother were likely to lead to particularly undesirable side-effects in the baby, such as hypotonia, jaundice and hypothermia. It is still used as an anti-convulsant in the treatment of severe pre-eclampsia.

### Hypnotics

There are a number of drugs which have been used to ensure some sleep in the early part of labour. They are all based on chloral hydrate and may be prescribed by midwives. Chloral hydrate is available as a syrup, but is unpleasant to take, and trichloryl (Trichlofos) and dichlor-alphenazone (Welldorm) are preferred.

### Barbiturates

Barbiturates were at one time popular both prior to and during established labour. One dose of barbiturate during labour is sufficient to decrease sucking frequency, sucking pressure and milk consumption by the baby. They were widely used at one time in the treatment of pre-eclampsia, but bed-rest is probably as effective.

### DRUGS ACTING ON THE UTERUS

Drugs acting on the uterus are of two types: those which stimulate its action (oxytoxics) and those which inhibit its action (tocolytics).

### Oxytoxics

Many substances have been used to stimulate uterine contractions, but only three remain in modern clinical practice. These are oxytocin, prostaglandin and ergometrine.

**Oxytocin.** Oxytocin is the hormone secreted by the posterior lobe of the pituitary gland, and is in some way, at present still unclear, involved in normal labour. The sensitivity of the uterus to oxytocin increases as pregnancy progresses, and it induces uterine contractions like those seen in normal labour. It has a mild water-retaining action, and if given in large doses, together with large quantities of 5% dextrose, can lead to fluid overload in the mother, with hyponatraemia. The infant can also be affected, and will also show hyponatraemia, which can cause convulsions. Oxytocin does not cause nausea and vomiting if given intravenously, but a bolus dose may cause a transient fall in blood pressure. An association between oxytocin and neonatal jaundice has frequently been suggested, but in clinical practice this appears to be both mild and short-lived.

**Prostaglandin.** Unlike oxytocin, which is a circulating hormone, prostaglandins are synthesized in the myometrium itself, and have an effect there before being rapidly destroyed. Stretching of the uterus is one stimulus to the synthesis of prostaglandins, and as with oxytocin, sensitivity of the uterus to prostaglandins increases as pregnancy advances. Two commonly used prostaglandins are prostaglandin $E_2$ and prostaglandin $F_2$ alpha. If given intravenously they are rapidly metabolized and so have to be given in large doses to produce the desired effect. There are other disadvantages to their intravenous use, so they are usually given as pessaries or vaginal tablets, or via the intra-amniotic or extra-amniotic route, to induce abortion. Prostaglandin $E_2$ may produce a rise in temperature.

**Ergometrine.** Ergometrine is an ergot alkaloid derived from a fungus. It induces a violent and often inco-ordinate spasm of the uterine muscle, rather than the rhythmic contractions of normal labour, and is therefore not suitable for induction or augmentation of labour. Its clinical use is limited to the prevention and treatment of uterine haemorrhage. It is often given in combination with oxytocin, as 'Syntometrine'; this is made up of 5 units of oxytocin, with ergometrine 0.5 mg. The main side-effect of ergometrine, especially if given intravenously, is vomiting. It also causes a rise in blood pressure, and is not given to patients with pre-eclampsia or essential hypertension.

### Tocolytics

Although there is much debate as to the the wisdom of inhibiting or attempting to inhibit premature labour, tocolytic drugs are widely used.

**The beta-adrenergic agents.** The drugs most often used are known as beta-adrenergic agents. The uterine muscle contains receptors which respond to sympathetic nerve stimulation, causing either contraction (alpha receptors) or relaxation (beta receptors) of the uterus. Drugs which act at these receptors have been developed. Drugs acting at the alpha receptors are not used to stimulate labour, since they cause uterine vasoconstriction and therefore reduced placental blood flow, and also tend to cause hypertension. The drugs stimulating the beta receptors have been designed to inhibit labour. Their use, however, may be complicated by tachycardia and hypotension, and patients so treated must be carefully monitored. The use of beta-adrenergic agents is generally contra-indicated in patients with cardiac or endocrine disease. They may interact with drugs used in anaesthesia, and patients receiving steroids to lessen the severity of respiratory distress syndrome in the baby may develop pulmonary oedema. The drug most commonly used is ritodrine (Yutopar). It is given initially as an intravenous infusion, and if labour is successfully inhibited, therapy may be continued orally. An alternative drug is salbutamol.

**Prostaglandin inhibition.** Many of the anti-inflammatory drugs used in the treatment of arthritis, such as aspirin and indomethacin, inhibit the synthesis of prostaglandins. Although these drugs would undoubtedly be effective in inhibiting uterine contractions, they are not suitable for this purpose, because they can cause serious side-effects in the baby, such as premature closure of the ductus arteriosus, with resulting damage to the heart and lungs.

As well as the specifically tocolytic drugs already described, many drugs inhibit uterine action as a side-effect. One example is halothane (see Chapter 3). Interestingly, ketamine relaxes the uterus in early pregnancy, but apparently has no effect on the myometrium nearer term. Adrenaline, which is another beta-adrenergic agent, also suppresses uterine activity, and if a local anaesthetic solution with adrenaline were used in an epidural block, this could prolong labour.

### SUGGESTED FURTHER READING

Central Midwives Board (1980) *Midwives' Rules.*
Chung, S. H. and Dickenson, A. (1981) The last piece in the puzzle. *Nursing Mirror,* 5th May.

Moir, D. D. (1980) *Obstetric Anaesthesia and Analgesia,* 2nd edn. London: Baillière Tindall.

Plantevin, O. M. (1973) *Analgesia and Anaesthesia in Obstetrics.* London: Butterworth.

Trounce, J. R. (1981) *Clinical Pharmacology for Nurses,* 9th edn. Edinburgh: Churchill Livingstone.

# 11 *Inhalational Analgesia*

Inhalational analgesia continues to provide many women with satisfactory pain relief in labour. Many women, both primigravidae and multigravidae, now benefit from epidural analgesia, and an increasing number will undoubtedly do so in the future. However, some women are resistant to the idea of an epidural block for a variety of reasons, and, of course, epidural block may not be available or may be contra-indicated (see Chapter 12). Inhalational analgesia is ideal for the woman who only requires pain relief at the end of the first stage of labour and who is anxious to remain ambulant for as long as possible. Inhalational analgesia may be administered by the midwife under the rules of the United Kingdom Central Council for Nursing, Midwifery and Health Visiting. These are:

FOR ENGLAND AND WALES
RESTRICTIONS ON ADMINISTRATION OF INHALATIONAL ANALGESICS

A practising midwife shall not, except on the instructions and in the presence of a registered medical practitioner, administer an inhalational analgesic to a patient unless:

She is satisfied from an examination of the patient by a registered medical practitioner during pregnancy that there is no contra-indication to the administration of the analgesic.

She has either before or after registration, received at a training school approved by the Board for the purpose, instruction in the essentials of obstetric analgesia.

A practising midwife shall not administer an inhalational analgesic by the use of any type of apparatus unless:

That type of apparatus is for the time being approved by the Council as suitable for use by midwives, and —

Where the Council so directs in relation to certain types of apparatus, the type of apparatus has been inspected and approved by or on behalf of the Council, within such period before the date of administration as the Council may determine, as fit for use by midwives, and a certificate to that effect, signed on behalf of the Council, is in the possession of the body or person by whom the apparatus is held.

RESTRICTION ON ADMINISTRATION OF ANAESTHETICS

Unless special exemption is given by the Council to enable a particular hospital to investigate new methods, a practising midwife must not administer any anaesthetic otherwise than on the instructions and in the presence of a registered medical practitioner.

NORTHERN IRELAND AND SCOTLAND

See general rules quoted in Chapter 10.

The Council rules pertaining to record-keeping and the inspection of equipment when requested also apply to the area of the midwife's responsibilities in the administration of inhalational analgesia.

Consideration will be given in this chapter to the use of nitrous oxide/oxygen, trichloroethylene (Trilene) and methoxyflurane (Penthrane).

## NITROUS OXIDE AND OXYGEN (ENTONOX)

Nitrous oxide is an anaesthetic gas (see Chapter 3) which, in a 50% mixture with oxygen, has analgesic rather than anaesthetic properties. When premixed with 50% oxygen it is known as Entonox; it is manufactured and supplied by BOC in a blue cylinder with a blue and white 'shoulder'. 'Gas and air', a term still wrongly applied to Entonox, was also a 50 : 50 mixture containing nitrous oxide, but mixed with room air rather than with oxygen. Because air contains 21% oxygen, a 'gas and air' mixture gave the patient only 10.5% oxygen, and so the days of 'gas and air' analgesia are often referred to nowadays as the era of hypoxic analgesia. Nitrous oxide was given in this way from the early 1930s until the final withdrawal of all 'gas and air' apparatus by the CMB in 1970. Despite its hypoxic properties, hundreds of mothers and babies appear to have emerged unscathed from this period. Dr Tunstall, an Aberdeen anaesthetist, mixed nitrous oxide and oxygen in equal proportions in one cylinder in 1962.

Entonox gives analgesia within 20 seconds if used correctly, and has its maximum effect after about 50–60 seconds. It is excreted rapidly by the lungs. Prolonged inhalation would lead to unconsciousness and this is why the principle of self-administration is so important. Entonox apparatus is fitted with both a reducing valve (see Chapter 3) and a 'demand valve'. This means that the gas does not flow, but has to be inhaled by a positive effort on the part of the patient. The patient takes it for herself as she feels the need, and because she holds the mask herself, she will drop it if she begins to feel sleepy. There are no side-effects unless administration continues over a long period, and the higher percentage of oxygen is likely to be beneficial to both mother and fetus.

The gas mixture is odourless, and any unpleasant smell arises from the tubing and mask. It is not explosive, though it does support combustion. Nitrous oxide is heavier than both air and oxygen, and this is relevant to the storage of cylinders.

**Entonox Equipment**

Entonox is administered from a piped supply in many modern units and, where this does not exist, from individual cylinders in transportable stands. A piped supply has its source in a 'manifold room', where large cylinders containing 5000 litres of gas are connected to the system of pipes which transport gas to each outlet. The reducing valve is situated on top of each cylinder or bank of cylinders, and there is a demand valve at each outlet point. From the outlet point, the equipment required is a length of black corrugated 'elephant tubing', an angle piece, an expiratory valve, and a face mask or mouth piece. The angle piece and expiratory valve may be combined or separate.

An individual Entonox cylinder which is transported to the patient's bedside as required has its reducing valve, demand valve and a contents gauge on top. The whole of this unit connects to the cylinder neck with a non-interchangeable pin-index system like that used with the other medical gas cylinders (see Chapter 2). The contents gauge gives an indication of the amount of gas remaining in the cylinder, just as it does in an oxygen cylinder. Attached to the cylinder in some way is a cylinder key (Fig. 11.1). A length of black corrugated 'elephant tubing' is also required and, again, an angle piece incorporating an expiratory valve, connecting the tubing to the face mask or mouthpiece.

Before use, the cylinder is opened, using the cylinder key, and the contents gauge is checked, before the cylinder is taken to the patient's bedside. Some patients may object to inhalational analgesia on the grounds that they fear feeling claustrophobic or suffocated. The use of a light mask, such as the Ambu mask, may be helpful here, but the mouthpiece designed by Dr Rosen in Cardiff may be more acceptable.

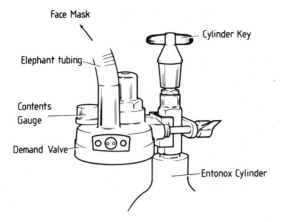

**Fig. 11.1** An Entonox cylinder and fitting, which includes both a pressure-reducing valve and a demand valve. The fitting is attached by means of a pin-index system (see Chapter 2).

This is a small plastic device, which the patient places between her lips and then sucks to inhale the gas. The expiratory valve is still incorporated in the circuit, so that she keeps the mouthpiece in position throughout her contraction.

### The Lucy Baldwin Apparatus

Lucy, Countess Baldwin, was the founder of the Anaesthetics Appeal Fund of the National Birthday Trust, committed to improving standards of care and safety in childbirth. The apparatus named after her is a modified dental anaesthetic machine, easily transportable, which carries two cylinders each of nitrous oxide and oxygen; the gases are in separate cylinders so that the ratios may be varied. It is approved by the CMB of Northern Ireland for use by unsupervised midwives under the usual provisos, as long as the ratio of nitrous oxide : oxygen is set at 50 : 50. It does not incorporate a demand valve, but the gas actually flows, so that anaesthesia is a real possibility. The ratio may be set as high as 70 : 30, but may only be used by a doctor when so set. A locking device must be released to allow delivery at a ratio of 80 : 20. A safety mechanism shuts off supply of one gas if the other fails to flow, and delivers room air to the patient. If required, in an emergency, the apparatus may be used to deliver oxygen only. One cylinder of each gas should obviously be a full one, and empty cylinders should be changed immediately.

**Care of Cylinders**

Entonox is a stable mixture except at temperatures of −7°C (19°F) or lower. In extreme cold the two gases will separate. Nitrous oxide is heavier than oxygen, and if cylinders are stored vertically, they may contain almost pure oxygen at the top and pure nitrous oxide at the bottom. For this reason, it is recommended that cylinders be stored horizontally at temperatures above −7°C. If cylinders have been stored horizontally, separation of the gases will lead to a mixture of uncertain ratio, but the administration of pure nitrous oxide is unlikely. After storage at low temperatures, it is recommended that cylinders should be kept in a room with a temperature of not less than 10°C for two hours. The cylinder is then inverted at least three times before use. The cylinder may be warmed by placing it in warm, not hot, water for 5–10 minutes, but the danger here is that water may get into the valve. Large cylinders containing 2000 or 5000 litres of gas and used as the gas source for a piped supply clearly cannot be inverted to ensure mixing of gases before use. It is therefore recommended that these should be stored horizontally at a temperature of between 10°C and 45°C for a minimum of 24 hours before use.

**Technique**

At most ante-natal preparation classes inhalational analgesia is discussed, and women are given the opportunity to try it out. This should make it seem less alarming when the time comes to use it in labour.

The principle of self-administration should first be explained simply to reassure the woman that she may take just as much as she requires and that she will not become unconscious. She should be reassured that any dizzy or detached feelings will pass off quickly, and are no cause for alarm. The fact that she obtains the gas on demand and that it does not flow continuously should also be explained. When she is in labour, she may be encouraged to try using the Entonox apparatus between contractions to get the feel of doing so. She should be told to fit the face mask firmly over her nose and mouth and to breathe steadily. 'Hyperventilation' or 'overbreathing' must be avoided. She then exhales, without removing the mask, and continues until she feels that the peak of her contraction has passed. She should start to use the 'gas and oxygen' as soon as she feels a contraction starting, so as to obtain maximum benefit. Her partner or companion may be very helpful in encouraging her in the use of inhalational analgesia, particularly if she becomes detached or very sleepy between contractions from the combination of narcotics and inhalational analgesia. Her partner may be shown how to palpate her contractions, or to observe them on the cardiotocograph and to guide the patient in recognizing their onset and commencing inhalational analgesia promptly. Some patients expect total analgesia and are dismayed to find that they do not obtain complete relief. Some women will find the sensations produced by Entonox unpleasant, particularly when combined with narcotics, while others will find them quite acceptable. Analgesia from Entonox reaches a peak within 50–60 seconds, but when inhalation ceases, nitrous oxide is rapidly excreted via the lungs. Attempts have therefore been made to maintain a low level of nitrous oxide within the body by administering Entonox via a nasal catheter using a continuous flow at a rate of 5 litres/minute. The background analgesia so obtained was augmented by inhalation in the usual way (though with a mouthpiece rather than a face mask) during contractions. No undesirable side-effects on either mother or fetus were described, and analgesia was improved, but the nasal catheter was, understandably, not well tolerated, so that the technique has not been further developed or become widely used.

## TRICHLOROETHYLENE (TRILENE)

This is a volatile agent. It comes in liquid form, and its vapour, transported in a carrier gas, acts as an analgesic or anaesthetic agent (see Chapters 2 and 3). It has a characteristic sweet smell which some women dislike.

For the purposes of obstetric analgesia, trichloroethylene is used in a vaporizer which utilizes room air as the carrier gas. The Central Midwives Board has approved two trichloroethylene inhalers, the Tecota Mark 6 and the Emotril Automatic. Production of the latter has now ceased, but there are still models in circulation. Both devices incorporate a temperature-compensating mechanism, so that the evaporation rate of the fluid is not significantly altered by room temperature, and they also have only two concentration settings — 0.35% and 0.5%. Administered at these concentrations, trichloroethylene has minimal side-effects, though drowsiness and perhaps some confusion and lack of co-operation may result from prolonged inhalation. Other inhalers have been designed, but as they do not incorporate these safety features, they have not been approved by the CMB for use by unsupervised midwives.

The Tecota Mark 6 (Fig. 11.2) and the Emotril are both neat, compact devices, fairly easily transported and easy to use. Each has a filling port leading to a sump where the fluid is soaked up by special wicks. As the patient inhales, air is drawn into the inhaler and through to the vaporizing chamber, where it picks up vaporized trichloroethylene, carrying it on through the circuit to the patient. The patient circuit is similar to that on the Entonox apparatus, consisting of a length of black 'elephant' tubing, an angle piece with an expiratory valve, and a face mask or mouthpiece. Where the elephant tubing leaves the inhaler, there is a one-way valve which prevents expired air from re-entering the vaporizing chamber. On the side of the inhaler is the concentration setting marked 'min' and 'max' (0.35% and 0.5%). An 'oxygen-enrich-ment device' is available for the Tecota Mark 6, so that extra oxygen may be drawn through as part of the carrier gas. The device fits over the top of the inhaler. A small 'window' near the filling port shows a fluid level, which gives a guide to the quantity of fluid trichloroethylene present in the sump. Like the vaporizer on the Boyles machine (Chapter 2), the inhaler should not be overfilled or underfilled, but a fluid level should always be visible in the 'window'.

Trichloroethylene is not used in a closed anaesthetic circuit as it may react with the soda lime used to absorb carbon dioxide from rebreathed gases, and form toxic fumes. If an obstetric patient requires a general anaesthetic after receiving trichloroethylene analgesia in labour, the anaesthetist should be informed that trichloroethylene has been used.

## METHOXYFLURANE (PENTHRANE)

Methoxyflurane is a substance similar to trichloroethylene in terms of both its chemical and its analgesic properties, though the general consen-sus of opinion seems to be that it is a more effective analgesic than either Entonox or trichloroethylene. It is administered via the Cardiff inhaler, which is very similar in appearance and design to the Tecota Mark 6. The Cardiff inhaler is green, while the Tecota Mark 6 is grey in colour. Methoxyflurane is delivered in a concentration of 0.35% only, which gives adequate analgesia, while a greater concentration often leads to excessive drowsiness. The Cardiff inhaler therefore has no alter-native concentration setting, but delivers a fixed rate of 0.35% methoxy-flurane in room air. It was approved by the CMB in 1971 for use by unsupervised midwives. The oxygen-enrichment device may also be used with the Cardiff inhaler.

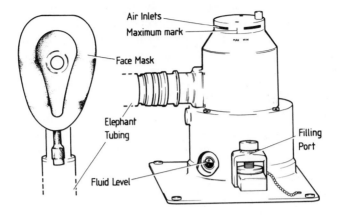

Air Inlets

Maximum mark

Face Mask

Elephant
Tubing

Fluid Level

Filling
Port

**Fig. 11.2** A Tecota Mark 6 inhaler for use with trichloroethylene.

In addition to its analgesic properties, methoxyflurane may give a feeling of detachment and mild euphoria.

It is not generally recommended that either trichloroethylene or methoxyflurane be used for a prolonged period, since both tend to have a cumulative effect in mother and fetus. They are therefore most useful in a short, painful labour. Unlike Entonox, their analgesic action reaches its peak after inhalation through two or three contractions, and neither substance is completely eliminated between contractions, so that a background analgesic effect is obtained. This cumulative effect gradually builds up, and in the case of trichloroethylene, it may be appropriate to reduce its concentration when analgesia is effective. The self-administration principle is important here, since the patient will reduce her intake when she needs less analgesia, and the levels of the agent within maternal and fetal tissues will then fall slightly. The CMB requires that all three inhalers, the Tecota, the Emotril and the Cardiff, be inspected annually on its behalf by the British Standards Institute, and that a certificate be issued to this effect. Responsibility for ensuring that this is done rests with the hospital concerned or with the individual midwife in domiciliary practice.

The use of inhalational analgesia has declined considerably with the introduction of epidural services and earlier intervention in abnormal labours. By far the most commonly used agent in the UK is Entonox, and it can be offered at any stage in labour. In the 1960s to 1970s inhalational analgesia was most often used only in the late first stage and the second stage. However, the use by midwives of trichloroethylene and methoxyflurane is still approved and taught in the UK, and can undoubtedly be invaluable for those practising in isolated areas.

## SUGGESTED FURTHER READING

Holdcroft, A. and Morgan, M. (1974) An assessment of the analgesic effect in labour of pethidine and 50% nitrous oxide in oxygen (Entonox). *Journal of Obstetrics and Gynaecology (British Commonwealth)* 81:603.

Moir, D. D. (1980) *Obstetric Anaesthesia and Analgesia,* 2nd edn. London: Baillière Tindall.

Central Midwives Board (1980) *Midwives' Rules.*

# 12 *Epidural Analgesia*

Epidural analgesia as a means of pain relief in labour has come into wide use over the past decade. An understanding of the procedure and its possible complications is essential for every midwife. Epidural, extradural or peridural analgesia may be performed in the lumbar or caudal regions, the former being much more common. Spinal or sub-arachnoid block is a different technique, and a comparison of the two procedures appears in Chapter 13.

### Anatomy
The epidural space is a small space surrounding the dura mater, the outermost layer of the meninges. The space measures approximately 4 mm between the ligamentum flavum and the dura mater in the lumbar region (see Figs. 12.1 and 12.2). It contains blood vessels and fatty tissue, and nerves entering and arising from the spinal cord pass through it laterally. The structures involved when approaching the epidural space are:

skin
a fat layer — usually minimal
supra-spinous and inter-spinous ligaments
the ligamentum flavum
the epidural space itself.

Lumbar epidural analgesia is usually instituted between lumbar vertebrae L1 and L2, L2 and L3, or L3 and L4. Occasionally the L4–L5 interspace may be used. The anaesthetist will palpate the spinous processes, using the iliac crests as landmarks in defining the inter-vertebral space he wishes to use (an imaginary line drawn between the iliac crests will pass through the fourth lumbar vertebra).

### Caudal Epidural Analgesia
Caudal analgesia is introduced via the sacral hiatus which lies between

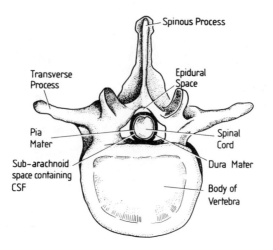

**Fig. 12.1** Cross section of the lumbar spine showing the anatomical structures involved in both lumbar epidural and spinal blocks.

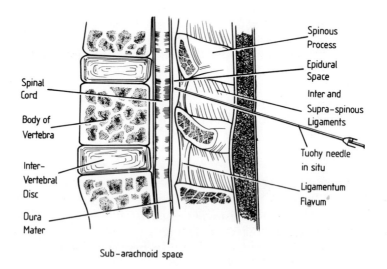

**Fig. 12.2** Sagittal section of the lumbar spine, with Tuohy needle in position.

the fifth sacral vertebra and the coccyx. Overlying the sacral hiatus is the sacrococcygeal membrane, and beyond this is the epidural space. The dural sac, containing cerebrospinal fluid (CSF), extends to the level of S2 (see Fig. 12.3).

Caudal analgesia may be performed with the patient in the prone, lateral or knee-chest position. The disadvantages of caudal block are:

Higher failure rate, usually due to anatomical variations, which are common.

Greater risk of toxicity because larger total doses of local anaesthetic are required.

The sacral nerves are blocked so that perineal sensation is lost, Ferguson's reflex (the reflex urge to bear down in the second stage of labour) is abolished, and a higher forceps rate results.

An epidural catheter may be introduced via the caudal route, and this will allow a higher block to be achieved. However, there is a risk of puncturing the dura mater as the catheter is passed (see Fig. 12.3).

Alternatively, a 'single-shot' technique may be employed, depending on the situation and on the patient's analgesic requirements.

## LUMBAR EPIDURAL ANALGESIA

### Preparation of the Patient
The procedure is explained to the patient, and opportunity given for questions or discussion. Her informed consent is then obtained in accordance with local policy. (Since written consent from a person who has received analgesic or narcotic drugs or who is distressed by pain may be considered invalid, this may not be thought necessary or desirable. The anaesthetist may then certify that he has explained the procedure fully to the patient and obtained her verbal consent).

The patient's blood pressure is measured and recorded at this stage.

An intravenous infusion is set up, and 500–1000 ml of crystalloid solution, such as Hartmanns solution, is infused. This reduces the risk of hypotension, which results from loss of peripheral vascular resistance caused by the degree of sympathetic block; this is secondary to the introduction of local anaesthetic solution.

Ephedrine must be readily available to treat hypotension whenever epidural analgesia is being instituted; ephedrine improves peripheral vascular tone without causing deterioration in the condition of the fetus.

Hypotension due to aortocaval occlusion must be avoided by the use of the full lateral position or a lateral wedge.

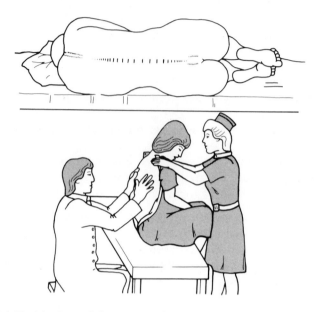

**Fig. 12.3** Positioning of the patient for epidural block: lateral and sitting. In both instances the spine is flexed.

The patient is now positioned either on her side or sitting (Fig. 12.3). If the lateral position is used, the anaesthetist will usually require the patient to lie on her left side, with her back at the edge of the bed or trolley, and perpendicular to it, that is, with her pelvic and pectoral girdles at 90° to the bed. The bed should have a firm mattress. Her thighs will need to be fully flexed, and her head should be down as far as possible so that her back is absolutely flexed. If the anaesthetist prefers to have the patient in the sitting position, the latter sits with her buttocks at the edge of the bed or trolley, with her feet resting securely on a stool or chair and with an assistant standing directly in front of her to support her shoulders. The patient then flexes her back.

**Equipment Required**

Sterile pack containing hand towel, gown, towel for the patient's back, and gauze swabs or sponges.

Sterile gloves.

Lotion or spray for cleaning the skin.

Syringe and needle for local infiltration.

Local anaesthetic solution.

Small disposable blade.

Tuohy needle — 16 or 18 SWG.

Epidural catheter — 16 or 18G as appropriate.

10 ml or 20 ml syringe which must run smoothly when the plunger is depressed; a glass syringe is usually used.

Antibacterial filter such as the Millex (Millipore).

Bacteriostatic spray such as povidone iodine if required.

Strapping such as sleek or a hypo-allergenic strapping.

Sterile ampoules of the local anaesthetic solution required and possibly also normal saline.

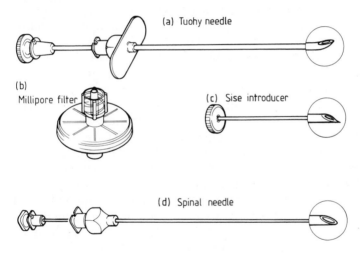

**Fig. 12.4** Equipment used for regional blocks: (a) Tuohy needle, (b) Millipore filter, (c) Sise introducer, (d) spinal needle.

The Tuohy needle is designed specifically for epidural use. It consists of a needle and stilette; it may be winged or plain. It has a bevelled end through which the epidural catheter may be directed into the space and upwards (or occasionally downwards) (see Fig. 12.4). This bevel is designed in such a way that the catheter, when passed through the needle, will emerge at a right angle. The needle tip is not sharp because of the risk of puncturing the dura mater and entering the sub-arachnoid space. The anaesthetist also has a better 'feel' of the tissues when he has a blunt needle.

Antibacterial filters are designed to filter out micro-organisms and particles of any kind, such as fragments of glass from ampoules.

Resuscitation equipment and drugs must always be readily available whenever an epidural block is performed.

**The Procedure**

The skin is cleaned and the back draped. Local anaesthetic is used to infiltrate the skin and deeper tissues. A small 'nick' is made in the skin with the blade, and the Tuohy needle with its stilette is introduced. It is advanced through the supra-spinous and inter-spinous ligaments to the ligamentum flavum which is very tough and strong. At this point the stilette is usually removed, and a syringe containing air or normal saline is attached. The Tuohy needle is now advanced very gradually, and the anaesthetist will test for 'loss of resistance' as he advances the needle. While the needle tip is in the ligamentum flavum, the plunger of the syringe cannot be depressed, that is, there is resistance. As the needle tip enters the epidural space, pressure will be atmospheric or negative; the plunger can then be depressed easily and air or normal saline can be pushed into the space without difficulty. Various devices are available for defining the change in resistance or pressure as the epidural space is entered. These include the Odom's indicator and the Macintosh balloon.

It is at this point of advancing the needle very gradually that some anaesthetists may prefer a 'winged' Tuohy needle to give them greater control over and 'feel' of the needle. The 'wings' are held with the thumb and first finger of each hand, while the second and third fingers may be braced against the patient's back in order to control the advance of the needle.

At this stage inadvertent entry into the sub-arachnoid space must be detected to prevent a 'total spinal'. Any leakage of cerebrospinal fluid (CSF) when the syringe is removed indicates that a dural tap has indeed occurred, and many anaesthetists prefer to test for 'loss of resistance' with air rather than with normal saline because they feel that the presence of CSF may not be detected if saline is used.

If no CSF or blood is seen, the epidural catheter is threaded through the Tuohy needle when the latter has been rotated so that the bevel is pointing in the required direction, that is, towards either the head or the feet. The anaesthetist will usually wait while the patient is having a contraction, during insertion of the Tuohy needle or the epidural catheter, particularly if she is distressed and restless.

The anaesthetist will note the depth at which the needle tip entered the epidural space; he will then be certain how many centimetres' length of catheter is lying in the epidural space, though it is not always possible to be certain of the direction in which it has travelled. The catheter is marked in centimetres. It is never withdrawn while the needle is still in position since there is a real danger of shearing off the end of the catheter on the inner edge of the needle bevel. The needle is removed from the epidural space over thê catheter, and the catheter is then withdrawn until the required amount remains in the epidural space (usually about 2–3 cm).

Many anaesthetists give a test dose of local anaesthetic solution as a routine; rapid onset of paraesthesia or anaesthesia of the legs and sudden hypotension will indicate that local anaesthetic solution has probably entered the sub-arachnoid space. The test dose, if given, will usually be  3–4 ml. If no adverse signs and symptoms are seen after five minutes, the remainder of the initial dose will be injected.

Positioning of the patient will depend both on the level of analgesia required and on the personal preference of the anaesthetist. The patient in early labour is likely to be placed in a wedged or full lateral position and may then be helped to turn onto her other side after five minutes, while for pain relief at the end of the first stage of labour or during the second stage, the patient may sit up during and after the injection of local anaesthetic.

Once the test dose has been given, the epidural catheter is strapped securely in place, usually straight up the patient's back, with the filter taped in front of the shoulder. The patient's blood pressure is measured and recorded five minutes after injection of the test dose. Once the main dose has been given, blood pressure will be measured and recorded as often as required by the anaesthetist, or in accordance with local procedure. The minimum interval for blood pressure recordings will usually be every five minutes for twenty minutes. The fetal heart rate should be monitored carefully throughout the procedure, particularly if any hypotension should occur. Local anaesthetic is not injected during a contraction, since venous congestion occurs as a result of the contraction. Congestion of the epidural veins reduces the available space in the epidural space, and so may cause increased spread of local anaesthetic solution, producing a high, patchy block. There may be a slight risk of puncture of an epidural vein if the needle or catheter is introduced into the space during a contraction.

## Drugs Used in Epidural Analgesia

The pharmacology of local anaesthetic drugs is discussed in Chapter 3.

The local anaesthetic drugs most commonly used for analgesia in labour are bupivacaine (Marcain) and lignocaine. Lignocaine has a rapid onset of action, but its effect is short-lived, so that if it were used over a period of time, the total dose would be considerable. Fetal and maternal toxicity may therefore be greater than that seen with bupivacaine, and so lignocaine (often 1.5%) has, until recently, most often been used as a 'single-shot' or final 'top-up' dose prior to operative delivery, suturing of the perineum or removal of a retained placenta. However, recent research has shown that effects on the fetus are not clinically significant.

Adrenaline is often added to local anaesthetic solutions because, producing local vasoconstriction, it reduces absorption into the blood, thereby reducing the incidence of toxicity; this also prolongs its effect (see Chapter 3). Bupivacaine, available in the UK as Marcain in 0.25%, 0.5% and 0.75% solutions, appears to affect the fetus very little.Analgesia, though slower in onset, is of longer duration than that obtained with lignocaine. Bupivacaine is available with added adrenaline, but this is not usually used in obstetrics because, unlike lignocaine with adrenaline, it does not produce lower blood levels, and furthermore, has an inhibitory effect on uterine contractions.

Weaker solutions of bupivacaine may be obtained by mixing with normal saline. Bupivacaine and lignocaine block sensory, motor and sympathetic nerves, so that the patient's legs may tingle or feel heavy or numb, or she may be unable to move them.

Local anaesthetic solutions are sometimes administered continuously via the Millex filter and the epidural catheter with the help of an infusion pump.This gives good analgesia but must be monitored carefully and adjusted as necessary.

Opiates may also be injected into the epidural space, but their analgesic effect in labour has so far been disappointing. Opiates block the opiate receptors in the pain pathway, but do not affect motor function. They give good post-operative pain relief and are often used following caesarean section. They may, however, cause respiratory depression, which may occur up to 12 hours after administration. The aetiology of this is as yet unclear. The patient's respiratory rate must therefore be observed carefully, particularly while she is sleeping, since such depression may occur insidiously, and be asymptomatic.

### Indications for Epidural Analgesia

Probably the most common indication for epidural analgesia is 'maternal request', as epidural services become established and as maternity care tends to become centralized in consultant units. While maternal reluctance remains an important contra-indication, certain obstetric conditions will increasingly result in medical recommendation of epidural analgesia. These include:

*Malpresentation or malposition.* Breech presentation was at one time regarded as a contra-indication because it was feared that laxity of the pelvic floor would inhibit descent of the breech, necessitating breech extraction with its associated increased morbidity and mortality. However, with the use of oxytocin, patients with a breech presentation generally do well with an epidural, and good analgesia for delivery is an undisputed advantage.

*Occipitoposterior position.* Again because of the laxity of the pelvic floor, rotation of the fetal head may be delayed and may ultimately have to be performed manually or instrumentally, but the long, distressing labour of a primigravida with an occipitoposterior position is undoubtedly helped by an epidural, though it may be difficult to alleviate backache completely.

*Pre-eclampsia.* Epidural analgesia is not regarded as a direct means of lowering raised blood pressure, though this may be a useful effect of the epidural. Rather, the analgesia afforded will prevent further rising of the blood pressure through pain and distress. Clotting studies must be seen to be normal in severe pre-eclampsia before epidural analgesia can be considered.

*Multiple pregnancy.* Good analgesia allowing any necessary manipulation and then prompt delivery of the second twin is generally thought to be a factor reducing morbidity and mortality.

*Diabetes mellitus.* Good analgesia for the mother with minimal effect on an already 'at risk' fetus is desirable in diabetic patients.

*Inco-ordinate uterine action.* In a labour where pain and distress are early symptoms with slow dilatation of the cervix, effective epidural analgesia appears to play a part in restoring uterine polarity.

*Premature labour.* Stress to the fetus caused by pressure on the soft, immature skull is thought to be reduced by epidural analgesia, with the associated reduction of tone in the pelvic floor. Again, minimal side-effects of analgesia on the neonate are seen.

*Maternal disease.* If the mother suffers from cardiovascular disease, for example, the stress of labour and delivery must be minimized, and elective forceps delivery may be planned.

**Contra-indications to Epidural Analgesia**
The main contra-indication to epidural analgesia is probably maternal reluctance, and better ante-natal education and more individual discussion and counselling could probably do much to dispel some of the misconceptions commonly raised in objection, and causing unnecessary fear. Other contra-indications include:

*Local or generalized infection.* Any risk of transmitting infection directly into the central nervous system is obviously best avoided.

*Any form of coagulation defect or abnormality.* A patient receiving anti-coagulant therapy is regarded as an unsuitable subject for epidural analgesia. Similarly, a patient who has suffered moderate or severe ante-partum haemorrhage or who has severe fulminating pre-eclampsia will usually be offered alternative forms of analgesia unless it is known that she has no coagulation defect. There is a risk that a coagulopathy could result in bleeding into the epidural space, with formation of a haematoma, which would exert pressure on the spinal cord. Such bleeding is obviously difficult to control.

Every patient is treated as an individual, and certain factors may be regarded as relative contra-indications.

*A scarred uterus.* This may be regarded as an absolute or a relative contra-indication. Some consider that the pain caused by the rupturing of a hysterotomy or previous caesarean section scar will 'break through' epidural analgesia, while others feel that it may not be detected if epidural analgesia is effective.

*Previous injury to or surgery on the back.* This may be a potential cause of difficulty with the institution of epidural analgesia, for example because of scarring and fibrosis as a result of surgery. Careful history-taking and examination by the anaesthetist will be necessary, preferably during pregnancy, before a decision can be made. Many such patients will wish not to have epidural analgesia because they will fear exacerbation or return of symptoms.

*Underlying neurological disease.* Problems such as disseminated sclerosis tend to become worse following pregnancy, and many anaesthetists feel that the epidural, if performed, may be cited as the cause of this, and that it is therefore best avoided because of the medicolegal implications as well as the patient's feelings.

## Complications

*Hypotension.* Because of the sympathetic block which accompanies sensory and motor block when local anaesthetic solutions are used in the epidural space, there is loss of peripheral vasomotor tone, and a fall in blood pressure may result. This may often be prevented by infusing 500–1000 ml of crystalloid solution before commencing the epidural — 'pre-loading'. Aortocaval occlusion must be prevented. Intravenous ephedrine may be required if hypotension is marked, and the patient should be turned onto her side, and oxygen administered at 6 litres per minute by face mask. The fetal heart rate must be closely monitored, and the obstetrician informed of any deterioration.

*Inadequate or unilateral analgesia.* This is an unfortunate, though not serious, situation which will be disappointing and often fairly distressing for the patient. The anaesthetist must be informed of any 'unblocked' segments, for example groin pain, since slight withdrawing of the epidural catheter and a further 'top-up' of local anaesthetic solution, with the patient appropriately positioned, may be all that is required. A unilateral block occasionally occurs for no obvious reason, and it is thought that some individuals may have a membraneous septum in the epidural space.

*Dural tap.* This occurs when the dura mater is punctured by either the Tuohy needle or, less commonly, the epidural catheter. Cerebrospinal fluid will leak out, and a 'spinal headache' commonly results. It is usual for the epidural then to be instituted at the adjacent interspace. The patient is kept lying flat, and an elective forceps delivery will be performed, so that the patient does not bear down and force further CSF out of the sub-arachnoid space. Management of the patient post partum will vary, but the anaesthetist will often want her nursed flat for a period of time. Some advocate encouraging the patient to lie prone as much as possible. The aim is to minimize leakage of CSF, which is the cause of the headache — a 'low pressure' headache. Many anaesthetists will inject normal saline through the epidural catheter following delivery, and then instil a litre or more of normal saline via an intravenous infusion set with the aid of an infusion pump over 24 hours. The aim of this is to maintain pressure in the epidural space and so discourage CSF leakage while the volume of CSF is restored to normal by the body. The intravenous infusion will be continued following delivery, and the patient will be encouraged to drink as much water as possible.

Analgesics are prescribed for the headache if it develops, and mild laxatives may be given to prevent constipation and straining in the early puerperium. If the 'spinal headache' develops and persists, the patient may be offered an epidural blood patch.

*'Bloody tap'.* This is the name given to inadvertent puncture of an epidural blood vessel, with consequent leakage of blood into the epidural catheter. Again the epidural will be recommenced and instituted at the adjacent interspace.

*Toxicity.* This usually results from intravascular injection of local anaesthetic solution; high total doses usually have to be given to cause a toxic reaction. Mild toxicity may cause tinnitus, dizziness or drowsiness. A major toxic reaction causes convulsions, but this is rare.

*A 'total spinal'.* This is considered last as it will rarely be seen. A 'total spinal' occurs when a 'dural tap' is undetected and local anaesthetic solution of a volume intended for the epidural space is injected into the sub-arachnoid space. Hypotension will usually occur immediately and dramatically. Sensation and motor function will be lost in the legs within minutes, and the patient's respiratory muscles will be paralysed shortly afterwards, though the apnoea may be partly due to the hypotension and circulatory collapse. It is for this reason that equipment for endotracheal intubation must be readily available whenever epidural analgesia is instituted. Artificial ventilation will be required until full respiratory function returns. If cardiovascular function and circulatory volume are quickly returned to normal and fetal distress does not ensue, labour may be allowed to progress normally. The patient will certainly not be the ideal candidate for caesarean section immediately after such a crisis! Unfortunately a 'total spinal' may cause convulsions, which are associated with a high incidence of placental separation, and in this event immediate caesarean section will be mandatory in the interests of the baby.

**Post-partum Discomforts and Problems**
The newly delivered patient has been through a major physiological event which is physically very demanding. Unless she was in a very fit state physically, she is likely to have various aches and pains to add to the considerable discomforts of perineal sutures and full breasts. Many of the symptoms commonly seen early in the puerperium are attributed, probably often unfairly, to the epidural block. Some women may feel vaguely guilty at having 'cheated' and escaped the pain of labour by having epidural analgesia, often as a last-minute decision in labour, and perhaps these women will more readily 'blame' the epidural block for their various discomforts.

*Backache.* Although this may be caused by the epidural block, particularly if more than one attempt was made to introduce the Tuohy needle, so causing slight local trauma, it is reasonable to suggest that backache is a likely sequel to any labour, particularly if several hours were spent on a hard labour ward bed or if the lithotomy position was used. It is likely to be a fairly short-lived symptom, and the patient may be reassured. Laxity of the pelvic ligaments may be a factor, just as it is in the backache common in pregnancy.

*Difficulty with micturition.* Again this is a common sequel to any labour, particularly after an instrumental delivery or a prolonged second stage, and it is caused by local trauma to the bladder neck and urethra. Certainly while the effect of the epidural block is still present, micturition may be a problem because of lack of sensation. Once the patient is fully mobile, with appropriate management of the problem she may be reassured that full function will return, and that the problem is probably physical rather than neurological in origin.

*Perineal pain.* This is often reported to be more severe following epidural analgesia. This may be due to lack of 'build-up' of pain during labour, and may involve endogenous opiate production. The second reason may be that because infiltration of local anaesthetic solution was not necessary at suturing, the sutures may be tight and therefore more painful.

*Headache.* 'Spinal headache' has already been discussed, and this is usually a quite characteristic frontal headache, often with associated neck stiffness. It is not seen following an uncomplicated epidural block. It seems reasonable to suggest that a headache may result from the patient's response to enthusiastic exhortations to 'push' in the second stage.

*Neurological symptoms.* Patients may sometimes complain of an area of anaesthesia or paraesthesia, often on the thigh. This is thought to be due to slight trauma to a nerve root during passage of the epidural catheter; it resolves in time. Other neurological symptoms are rare.

### Epidural Blood Patch

This will now be considered in more detail, since the midwife may be required to assist at this procedure. An epidural blood patch is an empirical treatment for 'spinal headache' which often results in dramatic improvement in the patient's condition. Some anaesthetists consider it an unreasonable risk because of the possibility of infection and because a spinal headache will resolve spontaneously after about a week. Others feel that the distress of the immobilized, photophobic, miserable patient should be alleviated if at all possible.

The procedure is normally performed by two people. One anaesthetist will locate the epidural space with a Tuohy needle, with full aseptic technique, while the other, again with full aseptic technique, wearing mask, gown and gloves, takes 10–20 ml of blood from a convenient vein. This blood is then handed to the first operator who injects it into the epidural space via the Tuohy needle. The needle is then removed, and the puncture site dressed.

Immediate relief is often felt. The patient may gradually sit up after about half an hour, and may then be fully mobilized. It is thought that the puncture site in the dura is sealed by a blood clot, and so energetic movement which might dislodge the clot is usually discouraged for 24 hours. Problems such as constipation or a cough may need to be treated. Any sign of infection should be reported promptly, but apart from this the patient may be up and about and start to care for her baby. The blood is reabsorbed into the system within days.

### Caesarean Section under Epidural Block

Generally speaking there is a certain resistance in the UK to the idea of undergoing surgery whilst conscious. Most individuals will automatically assume that having an operation involves a general anaesthetic. However, regional anaesthesia is being used more and more extensively, and is no longer reserved for patients such as the elderly bronchitic with an enlarged prostate or a fractured neck of femur, who is a 'poor risk' for general anaesthesia.

There are obvious advantages for the woman needing caesarean section; she will be able to see and handle her baby immediately in most cases. Many women who have already had a caesarean section under general anaesthesia recall that they felt a sense of detachment and unreality, uncertain as to whether events were dreams or not, for hours post operatively. Side-effects of general anaesthesia, though perhaps minor, are remembered as being unpleasant.

Caesarean section under epidural block offers the woman the opportunity to know as much as she wants to know about what is happening. She sees her baby immediately and feels that he or she is actually hers. She is likely to receive more effective post-operative analgesia, and so will be mobile more quickly, enabling her to care for her baby. Early mobility will also minimize post-operative complications such as deep vein thrombosis. Blood loss during caesarean section has been shown to be less under epidural block, and there are no recorded side-effects of any significance on the neonate, though opinion is divided on this question. The complications of general anaesthesia with the associated mortality and morbidity are avoided.

There are certain instances, however, where epidural block may not be the ideal means of anaesthesia. The contra-indications to epidural analgesia, relative or absolute, discussed earlier in this chapter, also apply here. Once again, uncertainty or reluctance should probably be regarded as a contra-indication. The very anxious woman, and probably one with any psychiatric disturbance, is not the ideal candidate. The woman being delivered of a very premature infant may be unduly distressed by the resuscitative measures employed and may not be able to see the baby for some while, which will add to her anxiety. Caesarean section for an anterior placenta praevia may result in considerable blood loss, and this may be regarded as a contra-indication to epidural block.

The woman having an epidural block for her caesarean section will be seen and examined by the anaesthetist in the usual way and will be prepared as if for general anaesthesia. She is told as much as she wants to know about the procedure itself and is given the opportunity to ask questions. She should be warned that she will not lose all sensation; she will feel pressure and movement as surgery proceeds, but will not feel pain. She may still feel apprehensive, and may be reassured that if she should feel at all distressed during surgery other means of pain relief will be used. Any unusual sounds, such as those arising from suction or diathermy equipment, should be explained. For the apprehensive patient, headphones with music of her own choice may be very helpful, since she can then dissociate herself from all that is going on until the baby is delivered. Sympathetic support and a hand to hold should always be offered. In an increasing number of centres, her husband may be allowed to be with her. Sensitive support and reassurance immediately before and during the operation will do more than anything else to allay anxiety.

Preparation of patient and equipment is as already described for epidural analgesia in labour. The block required is more extensive, and should affect the dermatomes (the skin areas supplied by the nerves) from S5 to T6, so that analgesia is effective over the entire abdomen and perineum. The patient will usually be unable to move her legs. To achieve this widespread block as well as muscle relaxation, a larger total dose of local anaesthetic solution (usually 0.5% or 0.75% plain bupivacaine) is required. This means that side-effects, such as hypotension, are more common and more marked. 'Pre-loading' with fluid intravenously is considered important as a preventive measure, and it is common to infuse at least 1000 ml, and perhaps 2000 ml, as the epidural block is commenced. Ephedrine and resuscitation equipment must be readily available. Positioning of the patient after injection of the local anaesthetic solution will vary with every anaesthetist's personal preference and with the progress of the epidural block in the individual patient. Sensation is usually tested by cold stimulus and pin prick, since these are appreciated by different sensory receptors. A patchy or unilateral block will be unacceptable, and a general anaesthetic may finally have to be given. For this reason, antacid therapy is usually given as a routine measure, just as it is given prior to planned general anaesthesia. A general anaesthetic may be given at any point during the operation, if necessary, though endotracheal intubation during surgery is obviously not ideal. All equipment and drugs for general anaesthesia must be checked and ready for use.

The patient's blood pressure and ECG are monitored during caesarean section, and it is common to ask her to breathe oxygen via a face mask until the baby is delivered. If the patient should feel any discomfort prior to delivery, she may be given added nitrous oxide in an analgesic ratio at the anaesthetist's discretion. After delivery of the baby, an opiate may be given intravenously for intra-operative discomfort, or an epidural injection of local anaesthetic solution or, again, an opiate may be given. The epidural block may be effective overall, but if traction is inadvertently applied to the peritoneum, abdominal packs are inserted with too much enthusiasm or the uterus is delivered onto the abdomen for suturing, this pain may 'break through' and cause distress. It is at these points that an otherwise satisfactory epidural block may need to be supplemented as described, and it is for these reasons that the block needs to be so profound and extensive. Another distressing side-effect is occasionally seen if liquor or blood spills into the paracolic gutter. This will often cause referred interscapular pain, which of course cannot be relieved by the epidural block. Occasionally patients will feel nauseated or will vomit as the peritoneum is being handled, and an intravenous anti-emetic may then be helpful. The distraction of having the baby to cuddle will also be helpful, and the patient is reassured that this is only a passing discomfort.

The majority of patients will find caesarean section under regional block a satisfying experience and will not suffer the various side-effects described.

Opiate analgesia via the epidural catheter gives very good post-operative pain relief. Morphine and diamorphine are commonly used. Opiates do not affect the motor nerves, so sensation and mobility of the legs will return to normal. The analgesia afforded is usually effective for several hours. Opiates used in this way do not cause hypotension, but systemic absorption may result in respiratory depression. The patient may not complain of any symptoms, but her respiratory rate should be observed and recorded post-operatively and after any further opiate 'top-ups'. When respiratory depression does occur, the patient's respirations become shallower and less frequent; her $PO_2$ then falls and she becomes hypoxic. She may appear to be sleeping during such an episode. Occasionally patients complain of itching, which may be severe and distressing, in which case no further opiate 'top-up' will usually be given.

**Nursing responsibilities**
Epidural analgesia is becoming firmly established as part of obstetric care, and so, in summary, the midwife's responsibilities will now be considered.

Preparation of the patient and equipment has already been discussed in some detail, and the midwife has a responsibility to ensure that she fully understands the procedure and its complications, so that she may give intelligent and efficient assistance with the institution of the epidural. She may find that the patient's questions and doubts are addressed to her rather than to the anaesthetist, and so she should be fully informed.

Once the epidural block has been established, the midwife will be primarily responsible for its management, in that she is the one providing the patient's immediate care. The anaesthetist takes the responsibility for the epidural block by initiating it, but he may delegate its maintenance to the midwife within certain limits. However, the epidural block remains the anaesthetist's contribution to the overall management of labour. He will prescribe 'top-up' doses of local anaesthetic solution and specify the position in which they are to be given, if this is in accordance with local policy and practice. If analgesia is patchy or ineffective, he should be informed, so that dosage or concentration of the local anaesthetic can be adjusted, or other measures taken. He may wish to be informed when full dilatation is confirmed and to prescribe differently, depending on the patient's particular requirements. Clearly the midwife is responsible for informing the anaesthetist of any complication such as hypotension, having herself instituted first aid measures, such as increasing the intravenous infusion rate, turning the patient onto her side and giving oxygen by face mask. Such measures will be laid down in local policy, and the midwife must be conversant with them.

The patient with an epidural block will lose bladder sensation, and so will be unaware of having a full bladder. She may be unable to pass urine, but a bedpan should be offered every two hours, just as it is in labour without an epidural block. If the patient is not able to pass urine, the bladder must be emptied by means of a catheter whenever appropriate.

**Management of the Second Stage of Labour**
The midwife should ascertain the wishes of the obstetrician and anaesthetist if she is uncertain as to how the second stage of labour is to be managed. A great deal of debate goes on over this, but current thinking

tends towards continuing to 'top-up' epidurals at full dilatation, albeit with a weaker solution if this seems appropriate. The ideal situation is one where Ferguson's reflex is present, and the woman feels the urge to bear down, but is still pain free. This is difficult to achieve, but the anaesthetist's aim is usually to maintain a reasonable level of analgesia, even if some sensation is permitted to return. In many labours under epidural block, there may be no cervix felt on examination, but the patient may feel no urge to bear down, and there may be no clinical signs of full dilatation. With good contractions, and a satisfactory fetal heart rate on cardiotocograph, labour may be left to progress until the head distends the perineum, and the woman feels the urge to 'push'. She is ideally nursed sitting upright during this 'latent' phase of the second stage. Encouraging pushing at this stage appears to achieve little apart from exhausting and discouraging the patient. Once descent of the head is seen, the patient is likely to want to push, or else will probably be able to do so effectively even in the absence of Ferguson's reflex if given appropriate instruction and encouragement. Allowing epidural analgesia to wear off completely at full dilatation, having kept the patient pain free during the first stage of labour, seems barbaric and unnecessarily distressing, since she will have had no build-up of pain (and probably also of endogenous opiates, though this is not fully understood as yet). Many anaesthetists feel that this practice results in higher incidence of forceps delivery than does the 'topping-up' of epidurals at full dilatation. A further reduction in forceps delivery rates has resulted from the move away from a slavish adherence to time limits on the second stage of labour. It is as a result of this line of thinking that the second stage of labour is sometimes sub-divided into the passive or latent phase and the active phase. While the fetal heart rate remains satisfactory, it is the active 'pushing' phase where time limits may be brought to bear in the absence of reasonable progress. Clearly the second stage of labour cannot be allowed to continue for hours, but more women now have the satisfaction of spontaneous vaginal delivery as a result of this broader approach.

## Care Following Delivery

The epidural catheter is normally removed following delivery. The patient lies on her side, with her spine flexed, and the catheter is withdrawn. The catheter is inspected before it is discarded, and if there is any doubt as to whether or not it is intact, the anaesthetist concerned should be informed and the catheter saved for his inspection. A small, dry dressing is applied to the puncture site. The intravenous infusion is normally discontinued following delivery, unless specific instructions are given to the contrary. The patient remains in bed until full sensation returns, and may then be fully ambulant. Any of the problems and discomforts already discussed should be reported to the doctor and symptomatic treatment and reassurance given as necessary.

**The 'Topping-up' of Epidural Blocks**
The United Kingdom Central Council for Nursing, Midwifery and Health Visiting makes the following statement:

"The Council would raise no objection to an experienced midwife undertaking the topping-up procedure (not the primary dose through the catheter) in the maintenance of an epidural block, providing the following safeguards are observed:
(a) that the ultimate responsibility for such a technique should be clearly stated to rest with the doctor,
(b) that written instructions as to the dose should be given by the doctor concerned,
(c) that in all cases the dose given by the midwife should be checked by one other person,
(d) that instructions should be given by the doctor as to the posture of the patient at the time of injection, observation of blood pressure etc., and measures to be taken in the event of any side-effect,
(e) that the midwife be thoroughly instructed in the technique so that the doctor is satisfied as to her ability."

The CMB for Scotland has permitted midwives to 'top-up' epidurals since 1978, with the provisos that individual hospitals should be approved by the CMB and that midwives should hold a 'certificate of competence' once suitably trained. Hospitals applying for approval were to have a fully established epidural service, with a resident anaesthetist available day and night, and with the service supervised by a consultant anaesthetist.

These statements of policy make it clear that this extension of the midwife's role does not relieve the anaesthetist of the ultimate responsibility, having delegated this particular task to her. However, every midwife will recognize her responsibility, as a professional person, to ensure that she is competent to carry out this task. If she is uncertain of any aspect of the task, she must seek further tuition. In undertaking the 'topping-up' of an epidural block she is tacitly stating her competence to do so.

## SUGGESTED FURTHER READING

Bromage, P. R. (1978) *Epidural Analgesia.* Philadelphia: W. B. Saunders.

Central Midwives Board (1980) *Midwives' Rules.*

Crawford, J. S. (1978) *Principles and Practice of Obstetric Anaesthesia,* 4th edn. Oxford: Blackwell Scientific Publications.

Hoult, I. J., Maclennan, A. H. and Carrie, L. E. S. (1977) Lumbar epidural analgesia in labour: relation to fetal malposition and instrumental delivery. *British Medical Journal,* 1:14.

Moir, D. D. (1980) *Obstetric Anaesthesia and Analgesia,* 2nd edn. London: Baillière Tindall.

Potter, N. and Macdonald, R. D. (1971) Obstetric consequences of epidural analgesia in nulliparous patients. *Lancet,* 22nd May:1031.

# 13 *Other Regional Blocks*

**Spinal Anaesthesia**

Spinal or sub-arachnoid analgesia has not enjoyed great popularity in the UK over the past few years, despite its wide use in the USA. This has largely been because of the feared risk of neurological problems and because of the commonly resulting 'spinal headache'. However, neurological sequelae are thought to have often been caused by chemical contamination of the local anaesthetic solution. Ampoules stored in phenol or other strong antiseptic or sterilizing fluids may have had micro-cracks in the glass, resulting in contamination of the contents. Better packaging and sterilizing techniques (ampoules are autoclaved today) should eliminate this problem. The use of fine spinal needles significantly reduces the incidence of post-spinal headache.

Spinal block has the advantages of producing good analgesia quickly; the technique is relatively simple, and the failure rate is low (Table 1). Analgesia may often be more profound and effective than that produced by epidural analgesia, but a continuous or intermittent technique is not generally thought practicable or desirable, though it has been performed and described. A 'single-shot' technique is therefore usually employed. Spinal analgesia is often useful in the second stage of labour for forceps or breach delivery, when epidural analgesia has not been used for some reason, or following delivery, for removal of a retained placenta.

The patient is prepared in much the same way as for the setting up of an epidural block. Spinal anaesthesia may be performed with the patient in the sitting or lateral position. The solution used is usually hyperbaric or 'heavy'; that is, it has a higher specific gravity than cerebrospinal fluid. Gravity will therefore affect the spread of the local anaesthetic, and positioning of the patient as it is injected determines the block achieved. Most of the local anaesthetic solution will have 'fixed' after 3–4 minutes and the block will be established, so that moving the patient after this time will not affect the block unduly, though the anaesthetist should be consulted before the patient is put into a lithotomy or head-down position.

Table 1. A comparison of epidural and spinal block

|  | *Epidural* | *Spinal* |
|---|---|---|
| Placement of local anaesthetic | Into the epidural space — no CSF | Into the sub-arachnoid space, i.e. into CSF |
| Total doses | Anything from 4 to 25 ml or even more | From 0.5 to 2.0 ml |
| Needle size | Usually 16G or 18G | Usually 22G, 25G or 26G |
| Onset of action | May be 15–20 minutes depending on local anaesthetic solution used | Rapid — occurs within minutes |
| Duration of action | Variable — continuous or intermittent technique with epidural catheter possible | 'Single-shot' technique usually employed |
| Risk of hypotension | Considerable unless intravenous fluid 'pre-load' given | Considerable unless intravenous fluid 'pre-load' given |

*The equipment* required includes:
   solution for cleaning the skin
   sterile 'spinal' towel
   local anaesthetic solution, syringe and needle for skin infiltration
   an introducer, such as the Sise introducer (see Fig. 12.4) or a cream 'drawing-up' needle
   a spinal needle, usually 22G, 25G or 26G (see Fig. 12.4)
   a 5 ml syringe containing the spinal anaesthetic solution
   a spinal filter or a Millex filter
   a small dressing for the puncture site

*The Procedure*
The anaesthetist scrubs and dons sterile gown and gloves. With the

patient in the required position, he cleans, drapes and infiltrates the skin. The introducer is used to pass through the skin and into the ligamentum flavum, as the fine spinal needle would be likely to bend or break if it were passed through these tough tissues. The spinal needle is then passed through the introducer, into the epidural space and through the dura mater into the sub-arachnoid space. The anaesthetist often senses a 'give' as the needle penetrates the dura mater. Leakage of CSF occurs gradually with the fine gauge needles (25G and 26G), but may be seen with the larger needles (22G and larger), when a drop is seen at the needle hub. The local anaesthetic solution is then injected. There is a slight possibility of drawing up minute glass fragments with the local anaesthetic solution, and 'spinal filters', which look like hypodermic needles, are available. Alternatively, the solution may be filtered through a Millex epidural filter. Once the local anaesthetic solution has been injected, the introducer and needle are withdrawn, and a small dry dressing is applied to the puncture site.

It is important that the local anaesthetic solutions for preparatory infiltration and for the spinal block itself should not be confused. A 5 ml syringe may therefore be used for the latter, though only a small volume of solution is required.

*Drugs Used*
Cinchocaine (Nupercaine) and mepivacaine (Carbocaine) both in dextrose solution to render them hyperbaric, are currently available in the UK. Lignocaine and amethocaine (Tetracaine or Pontocaine) are used outside the UK but have so far not been approved by the Committee on the Safety of Medicines (amethocaine may be obtained from certain NHS pharmacies which make it). Bupivacaine 0.5% has recently received this approval; it is isobaric rather than hyperbaric, so that volume of solution used rather than positioning of the patient determines the level and extent of the block achieved. The dosage of any of these drugs varies between 0.5 ml and 2 ml depending on the extent and type of the block required.

Barbotage is the name given to the mixing of CSF and local anaesthetic solution by injection, aspiration and re-injection. This allows a higher block to be obtained with smaller volumes of local anaesthetic solution, but it is rarely, if ever, used in obstetrics.

As with injection of local anaesthetic solution into the epidural space, it is usual to inject between uterine contractions because of venous congestion. Turbulence of CSF during contractions and a rise in CSF pressure may result in a more widespread and perhaps less effective block.

As with epidural analgesia, hypotension may occur as a result of sympathetic block. It will occur almost immediately, as does the analgesic effect. An intravenous infusion is normally in progress if a sub-arachnoid block is to be performed. Motor block is often profound, and patients may dislike this feeling. Bladder sensation is lost.

It may be several hours before sensation returns completely to normal following spinal block. Nupercaine has the longest duration of action, and lignocaine probably the shortest. It has been usual to keep patients lying flat for 12–24 hours following spinal blockade, in order to minimize the frequency and severity of post-spinal headache, but with the advent of finer gauge needles, the value of this practice is being questioned. Certainly there are obvious disadvantages to the newly delivered woman if she has to remain in bed, and some may be very disappointed by this restriction; at the same time, pregnant and newly delivered women appear to be more prone to spinal headaches than their non-pregnant counterparts. The anaesthetist's wishes must be ascertained and carried out as far as after-care is concerned. The patient must certainly remain in bed until the motor block has worn off completely. A high fluid intake is normally advocated; this may be via the intravenous route or orally or both. Again this is to minimize post-spinal headache by ensuring adequate fluid levels to enable reconstitution of leaked CSF in the shortest possible time. Bladder care is important until the block has worn off. Impaired sensation may inhibit micturition, and retention of urine must be detected and treated. Contra-indications are the same as those to epidural block (see Chapter 12).

**Spinal Blocks Used in Obstetrics**
These are described according to the location and extent of the block.

*Saddle block.* This describes the type of block achieved by injecting local anaesthetic solution with the woman in the sitting position. Anaesthesia of the perineum and lower birth canal is obtained by blocking the sacral nerves, and this is suitable for low forceps delivery or suturing of the perineum. However, it does not allow any kind of uterine manipulation, such as that required for manual removal of a retained placenta.

*Low spinal block.* This type of block extends from T10 to S5; it gives motor and sensory block from the waist down, and so may be used for any type of operative delivery apart from caesarean section, for exploration of the uterus and for manual removal of the placenta. It is achieved by placing the patient in a sitting position for, say, 30 seconds, and then placing her supine with a lateral wedge. A low spinal block is not sufficiently extensive for caesarean section.

*Mid-spinal block.* This is the block required for caesarean section, and it extends from T6 downwards. Because it is so extensive, the risk of hypotension is considerable, but it seems likely to become more popular in the UK in the near future. Its advantage over epidural block is its rapidity of onset; it is also reliable and gives good muscle relaxation. Blood loss at surgery is reduced, as with epidural block.

**Paracervical Block**

Paracervical block has not enjoyed great popularity in the UK in the recent past though it has been widely used elsewhere.

The block is performed by injecting local anaesthetic solution into the lateral fornices in order to block the paracervical plexus. All the uterine nerves are involved in this plexus, so relief of first stage pain is obtained. However, analgesia of the vagina and perineum is not achieved, so that further analgesia, such as a pudendal block, will be required if operative delivery is necessary. Paracervical block is easily performed and does not necessarily require the skills of the anaesthetist. Analgesia may last for up to three hours, but this means that the procedure may need to be repeated. The uterine artery lies adjacent to the paracervical plexus, so that intra-arterial injection is a possible danger. This is one of the causes of the fetal bradycardia which may be seen and, indeed, perhaps of otherwise unexplained intra-uterine deaths that have been reported. This is the main reason, along with the wider availability of epidural blockade, for its now infrequent use.

*The procedure.* With the patient in the lithotomy position, and using aseptic technique, the obstetrician places the needle tip within the paracervical tissue. A guarded needle is used to prevent injection to a depth greater than 5 mm, though some recommend only 2 mm. Examples of such needles include the Kobak (Oxford) needle (Fig. 13.1) and the Iowa trumpet. After aspiration for blood, 5–10 ml of local anaesthetic solution, usually lignocaine 1% or bupivacaine 0.25%, is injected. It is common to wait for 5 minutes before the remainder of the dose is injected into the other lateral fornix. The risk of both maternal and

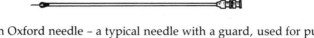

**Fig. 13.1** An Oxford needle – a typical needle with a guard, used for pudendal or paracervical block.

fetal toxicity is further reduced by dividing the total dose into four and injecting at two sites in each lateral fornix. Maternal pulse and fetal heart rates are observed in the meantime. It is possible to inject local anaesthetic solution into the myometrium or even into the fetus itself, and this will result in high fetal blood levels of local anaesthetic and fetal depression.

Because of the risk of fetal bradycardia it is not usual to use paracervical block in cases of fetal distress, prematurity or intra-uterine growth retardation.

**Pudendal Block**
This is another relatively simple regional technique used for operative vaginal delivery in the absence of other regional block and performed by the obstetrician. Local anaesthetic solution is injected to block the pudendal nerves, which supply the vagina, perineum and pelvic floor. The pudendal artery is adjacent to the pudendal nerve, and posterior to the pudendal nerve is the sciatic nerve. Again, a guarded needle is used to prevent too deep an injection.

*The procedure.* The transvaginal approach is usually used, though the transperineal approach may be used if the presenting part is very low. The ischial spines are palpated, and the sacrospinous ligament defined. The pudendal nerve lies directly posterior to the ligament, and the needle is passed through it near its point of insertion at the ischial spine. After aspiration for blood, up to 10 ml of local anaesthetic solution is injected, and the procedure is then repeated on the other side. It is usual to infiltrate the perineum as well.

Pudendal block has a fairly low rate of total success; good analgesia bilaterally is reported to be achieved in about 50% of patients. A fair degree of analgesia is probably achieved in a good proportion of the remaining 50%.

## SUGGESTED FURTHER READING

Bonica, J. J. (1972) *Obstetric Analgesia and Anaesthesia.* Berlin: Springer-Verlag.

Moir, D. D. (1980) *Obstetric Anaesthesia and Analgesia,* 2nd edn. London: Baillière Tindall.

Pearce, J. M. S. (1982) Hazards of lumbar puncture. *British Medical Journal,* 285:1521.

Ravindran, R. S., Vegas, O. J., Tasch, M. D., Cline, P. J., Deaton, R. L. and Brown, T. R. (1981) Bearing down at the time of delivery and the incidence of spinal headache in parturients. *Anaesthesia and Analgesia,* 60:524.

# 14 Resuscitation of the Newborn

As the paediatrician has become more involved in the care of the newborn baby in the delivery room, midwives now find themselves actively resuscitating the baby less frequently. However, resuscitation still remains an important part of the midwife's role, and it is vital that she should maintain these skills and feel confident in using them.

Of equal importance is the support and reassurance given to the parents. Even basic resuscitative measures can look extremely alarming, and both parents may be feeling tired and emotional. A simple explanation of what is likely to occur following delivery and the introduction of the paediatrician as another member of the caring team may do much to alleviate anxiety. When a baby requires more prolonged resuscitation, honest explanation and realistic reassurance must be given in as much detail as individual parents require. The baby should be given to them for a cuddle as soon as his or her condition permits.

An outline is given in this chapter of the principles and dangers involved in resuscitation of the newborn, and of the equipment required.

Mouth-to-mouth resuscitation has been known and described from ancient times, and still has its uses.

## Anticipation of Need
In considering the resuscitation needs of any baby and preparing to meet those needs, certain high risk groups can be identified. With fetal monitoring in labour, intra-partum hypoxia and fetal distress should be detected, and babies suffering from the after-effects of such symptoms are more likely to require active resuscitation at birth. Any obstetric complication, such as malpresentation, ante-partum haemorrhage, pre-eclampsia or instrumental delivery, may result in a baby requiring resuscitation, and fetal factors include prematurity and intra-uterine growth retardation. The mother who has received narcotic analgesia within the six hours prior to delivery may have a baby whose response to the stimulus of birth is sluggish. It is usual, in the major obstetric units

in UK today, to inform the paediatrician of the imminent delivery of all mothers in the above categories, so that he or she may be present. In any event, a full range of resuscitation equipment should be readily available, checked and in good working order, for all deliveries.

### Assessment

All babies are quickly assessed at birth, and the means of assessment in common use is the Apgar score. Dr Virginia Apgar was an anaesthetist in the USA, and her criteria for assessment are shown in Table 2.

Each factor scores 0, 1 or 2 — poor, fair or good — giving a maximum score of 10. The Apgar score is assessed at one minute after delivery, and usually thereafter at 5 and 10 minutes of age. It may be helpful to assess the baby's Apgar score immediately after birth, and in some centres it is also assessed at 2 minutes. In cases of severe depression it is assessed and recorded until satisfactory. In this way it can be used as a guide to progress during the period of resuscitation, particularly in retrospect. Like all such assessments it has its limitations, and observer variation and subjectivity can be considerable. In some centres, colour is disregarded, being thought less helpful and often a misleading factor, and the neonate is assessed on the first four factors. 'Apgar minus colour' is then recorded as 'A–C', with an optimum score of 8. Dr Apgar was careful to assert that resuscitation should commence at the earliest opportunity, and not at the one minute assessment.

The majority of babies born normally at term respond to the various stimuli of birth and require no active resuscitation. Thorough drying and wrapping in a warmed towel is often all that is required. Suction of the airway may lead to 'reflex apnoea', and should be performed only if really necessary.

### The Depressed Infant

The depressed, hypoxic infant requires prompt, appropriate treatment. Birth asphyxia is described in the following stages:

*Primary apnoea.* Here some respiratory effort is seen, but the baby may only gasp. Thrashing movements of the limbs occur. Spontaneous ventilation may be initiated by external stimuli at this stage, but the infant will rapidly become more hypoxic until the lungs are inflated and oxygenated. The heart rate falls. After a period of apnoea the baby will gasp for a few minutes and the heart rate may increase, but if

Table. 2. The Apgar scoring system

| | Absent | Less than 100 | More than 100 |
|---|---|---|---|
| Heart rate | 0 | 1 | 2 |
| | Absent | Gasping | Spontaneous respiration |
| Respiratory effort | 0 | 1 | 2 |
| | Limp | Some flexion of extremities | Active limbs flexed |
| Muscle tone | 0 | 1 | 2 |
| | No response | Grimace | Cry |
| Reflex irritability* | 0 | 1 | 2 |
| | Blue or pale | Body pink, extremities blue | Completely pink |
| Colour | 0 | 1 | 2 |

* In response to stimulation of foot, for example.

ventilation and oxygenation of the lungs are not achieved, secondary apnoea will ensue.

*Secondary or terminal apnoea.* In this stage the baby is severely hypoxic and hypercapnic. Bradycardia and hypotension are symptoms of circulatory failure caused by metabolism and therefore depletion of cardiac glycogen stores. Metabolic and respiratory acidosis increases rapidly. At this stage apnoea cannot be reversed by external stimuli, and unless hypoxia and acidosis are also reversed, the baby will die within minutes of the 'last gasp'.

The depressed baby may be in either of these two stages at delivery. If a hypoxic episode has occurred prior to delivery, the baby may already have passed through the stage of primary apnoea before birth, and be born in a state of secondary apnoea. Cerebral hypoxia, which may lead to irreversible brain damage in some infants, is then likely to be present, though such damage cannot be assessed at this early stage. At least 80% of infants born with Apgar scores of 0 or 1, who then survive, do not have a major handicap. Prognosis depends on subsequent events — in particular, assessment by means of the developmental 'mile stones'. Having said this, the newborn baby is better able to withstand hypoxia than the older child or adult. This is partly because the immature brain, unlike that of the adult, is able to metabolize ketone bodies anaerobically and so maintain itself. Fetal circulation will persist in perinatal hypoxia; 'shunting' of blood to the brain and heart occurs, giving a degree of protection from the worst effects of hypoxia. Peripheral vasoconstriction occurs and will further assist in this. When fetal circulation persists in this way, however, pulmonary artery pressure remains high, leading to increased 'shunting' of blood from right to left through the foramen ovale, as well as at the ductus arteriosus. Cerebral oxygenation is then less efficient than it is when the normal circulatory changes have occurred.

**Physiological Changes at Birth**
The physiological changes occurring at birth are partly dependent on the initial inflation of the lungs. Until this occurs, blood from the superior vena cava is 'shunted' through the foramen ovale, and the ductus arteriosus remains fully patent. When ventilation of the lungs does occur, full pulmonary circulation commences, with gaseous exchange taking place. Blood from the pulmonary vein enters the left atrium, and the raised left atrial pressure causes functional closure of the foramen ovale. Rapid initial but incomplete constriction of the ductus arteriosus is followed by gradual complete closure over a period of days. This constriction is thought to be due to raised oxygen tension in the arterial blood.

The fetal lungs are filled with fluid, which is a transudate and not amniotic fluid, though if the baby suffers a hypoxic episode before delivery and gasps, a mixture of the two is usually present. Drainage of this fetal lung fluid occurs from the baby's mouth after birth; it is aided by thoracic compression in the birth canal during the second stage of labour. Some of the fluid is absorbed through the alveoli and drained by the pulmonary lymphatics. Because this fluid is present in the alveoli, the initial expansion of the lungs requires greater pressure than is needed thereafter.

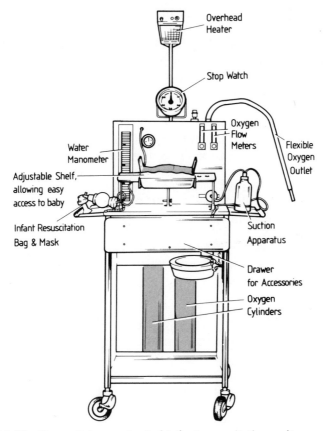

Overhead Heater

Stop Watch

Water Manometer

Oxygen Flow Meters

Flexible Oxygen Outlet

Adjustable Shelf, allowing easy access to baby

Infant Resuscitation Bag & Mask

Suction Apparatus

Drawer for Accessories

Oxygen Cylinders

**Fig. 14.1** The Resuscitaire — a typical infant resuscitation unit.

### Equipment Required

Infant resuscitation equipment is conveniently kept together in a transportable unit, such as the Resuscitaire (Fig. 14.1). This type of unit provides a working surface at a convenient height, with an overhead radiant heater, an oxygen source, suction equipment, and a drawer and shelves for storage of equipment. The working surface may be adjusted to give head-down tilt if required.

This equipment includes:

*Laryngoscopes.* At least two, checked and in good working order, with spare batteries and bulbs readily available.

*Neonatal endotracheal tubes and introducers.* Endotracheal tubes are usually disposable, and should be available in sizes 2.5 mm or 3.0 mm. Each tube should have its connector attached, and an introducer should be ready for use. Neonatal tubes commonly have a 'shoulder' near the distal end, to prevent too deep an insertion into the trachea.

*A neonatal resuscitation bag such as the Ambu or Laerdal bag.* These have an air inlet with a one-way valve, and a connection for tubing to the oxygen supply, an inflation bag, a safety valve to prevent over-inflation of the lungs, and can be connected either to a face mask or to the endotracheal tube. The proportion of oxygen administered via such a bag may be increased by covering the air inlet with the hand and by filling the bag with oxygen before use. Alternatively, the lungs may be inflated using only room air.

*Neonatal airways.* These should be available for babies with anomalies such as choanal atresia. Neonatal Guedel airways come in sizes 0, 00, and 000.

*Sterile suction catheters.* A selection, say 6FG, 8FG and 10FG, should be available so that suction of the mouth and oropharynx may be performed, or, if necessary, deeper suction can be performed via the endotracheal tube.

*Face masks.* These should be available in at least two sizes to ensure a good fit for any baby.

*'Silver swaddlers'.* These are wraps of silver foil, designed to prevent heat loss. They only conserve body heat already present, and will not warm an already hypothermic baby, but are useful for transporting very small or sick babies.

*Syringes, needles, spirit swabs, equipment for setting up a scalp vein infusion or inserting an umbilical catheter.* This consists of a sterile pack containing gown, towels and fine instruments; to this is added solution for cleaning the skin, a suitable cannula or catheter as required, and a fine silk suture if required. These procedures may occasionally need to be carried out before moving the baby.

*Drugs*

*Narcotic antagonists.* Usually naloxone (Narcan) — see Chapter 10. Other narcotic antagonists are nalorphine (Lethidrone) and levallorphan (Lorphan), but these are now less commonly used. Naloxone is given to the baby who is thought to be depressed as a result of narcotics given to the mother during labour. Naloxone is available for use with neonates in ampoules containing 0.04 mg per ml. A term baby may be given 0.04–0.08 mg intramuscularly, and will respond within 90 seconds if he was suffering from narcotic-induced respiratory depression.

*Sodium bicarbonate.* This has been used in the past to reverse metabolic acidosis, but is now thought to be of no value.

The oxygen source already mentioned may be a cylinder attached to the unit or the central piped supply. The oxygen usually has two outlets, controlled separately, each with its own flowmeter. The main outlet is used to give oxygen either through the endotracheal tube or by face mask. It is important that the baby's lungs should not be overinflated, particularly after the initial inflation, and a water manometer may be incorporated as a safety device. The oxygen tubing leading from the source has a side-arm situated in the manometer, which is mounted on the infant resuscitation unit. This side-arm leads down the manometer into the water to a depth of, say, 30 centimetres. If oxygen is then given at a pressure greater than 30 cm of water, or 2.9 kPa, the excess will bubble harmlessly through the water and out into the atmosphere. The blow-off valve on the resuscitation bag provides a further safeguard against excessive pressure. If such a bag is not used, then the IPPV tubing may simply incorporate a hole which is occluded by the operator's finger during inflation of the lungs and uncovered for exhalation, or a 'Y-piece' may be used. In this case oxygen flows through one arm of the Y-piece, and the other is occluded during inflation and again uncovered for exhalation. The second oxygen outlet, if present, may be used to blow oxygen gently onto the baby's face, to act as a stimulus. This has the advantage of enriching the air around the baby's nose and mouth with oxygen, but the disadvantage is that cold, dry gas may cause reflex apnoea. Some authorities disapprove of its use for this reason.

A stop-watch is usually mounted on the unit, so that progress may be monitored and the sequence of events recalled with reasonable accuracy.

**The Principles of Resuscitation**
These may be summarized as:
Prevention of cooling
Clearing of the airway
Inflation of the lungs

Hypothermia will add to the problems of the hypoxic baby. A fall in environmental temperature of 2°C below the thermoneutral range (32–34°C for a term infant) leads to a doubling of the baby's oxygen consumption. Thus, if the baby is asphyxiated the time taken to utilize his oxygen store is halved, so reducing his 'intact survival time' very significantly. Newborn babies do not maintain their body temperatures well, and all babies should be thoroughly dried as soon as possible after the moment of birth, and then be wrapped in a warm towel. The temperature of the delivery room should be at least 20°C, and preferably warmer. Frequently, a term baby will require no further stimulation than drying and wrapping, except perhaps minimal suction, and may then be left with his mother for a cuddle, to benefit from her body warmth. The head is an area from which significant heat loss may occur, and this should be borne in mind when drying and wrapping the baby.

The baby requiring active resuscitation must also be thoroughly dried, and the overhead heater, which should be switched on well before delivery, may then be used to minimize heat loss. It should be possible to partly wrap the body, although the chest needs to be visible, in order to observe any respiratory effort or to auscultate the heart or lungs. A silver swaddler, together with warmed blankets, may be useful, particularly for a small baby. Hypothermia in a small or sick baby will cause further depletion of glycogen stores, slowed metabolism and increased incidence of morbidity, as discussed in the preceding paragraph.

A chilled baby is nursed in an incubator, fed as soon as possible, by tube if necessary, and hypoglycaemia treated if it occurs. The baby's temperature is monitored; overheating must also be avoided.

The airway usually contains fetal lung fluid and amniotic fluid at birth. It may also contain blood or meconium. Prevention of meconium aspiration is very important, since this may block bronchioles and alveoli, being more viscous than the secretions mentioned. Compression of the chest may be helpful in delaying the first breath until suction of the mouth and oropharynx has been carried out, usually under direct vision with a laryngoscope. Suction should usually be minimal and gentle, since excessive use of a suction catheter may cause reflex laryngeal inhibition, which will delay the establishment of spontaneous respiration. However, when meconium is present in the trachea, suction must be sufficiently thorough to remove it completely.

When IPPV is performed via an endotracheal tube in an asphyxiated baby, it may be useful to pass a suction catheter down the tube prior to extubation and to perform gentle suction as the tube is withdrawn.

Positioning of the baby is important when attempting to resuscitate, since hyperextension of the neck may lead to airway obstruction. The placing of a small pad under the shoulders usually gives optimum positioning. The use of head-down tilt in order to aid drainage of secretions has been popular, but many paediatricians now feel that pressure from abdominal organs on the diaphragm may cause some respiratory embarrassment and prefer either slight head-up tilt or the horizontal position.

Because the stomach usually contains amniotic fluid, blood and mucus, many feel that it is helpful to empty the stomach by means of a nasogastric tube. Regurgitation of stomach contents will not then cause any airway obstruction and feeding is thought to be more readily established. In the presence of excessive mucus it is necessary to ascertain at an early stage whether or not the oesophagus appears to be complete. This is assumed to be the case if a nasogastric tube can be passed easily and if acid aspirate is then obtained, so ruling out the possibility of oesophageal atresia. Gastric aspirate may usefully be examined microscopically and cultured, for example, following prolonged rupture of the membranes, in order to identify any incipient or overt infection.

Inflation of the lungs in a baby who is not breathing spontaneously is carried out by intermittent positive pressure — IPPV. This may or may not involve the use of an endotracheal tube.

IPPV using a face mask may be given initially. The baby's chin is supported by the third and fourth fingers of the hand holding the mask, and the head is tilted back slightly in the position described as 'sniffing the morning air'! The aim is to maintain a clear airway and an air-tight fit of the mask upon the face. The bag is inflated about 40 times per minute. Abdominal distension will indicate inflation of the stomach; the chest should be seen to rise and fall with inflation, and the baby's colour should improve. If some respiratory effort does not ensue, then endotracheal intubation should be considered. Once some respiratory effort is seen, it is important not to inflate the baby's lungs out of sequence with his own attempts to establish a rhythm.

If the baby is severely asphyxiated, with an Apgar score of 3 or less, or if he shows no sign of respiratory effort, or resuscitative measures are not proving effective, then intubation is necessary. With the baby positioned as described, supine with the head just slightly tilted back, the laryngoscope blade is gently inserted. The laryngoscope is designed for use in the left hand, and the blade is passed along the tongue. When the epiglottis is seen as a small pink flap at the back of the tongue, the blade is slipped carefully underneath it, and lifted up. The glottis should then be visible as a small vertical slit. The cords are not as easily identified as they are in an adult, but if the baby gasps at this point, they may open, and the slit of the glottis becomes triangular. Once the glottis is seen, the endotracheal tube is introduced, using the right hand, and is passed through the glottis. If the glottis cannot be visualized, gentle cricoid pressure using just one finger very lightly may bring it into view. Once again, if inflation causes abdominal distension, oxygen is being blown into the stomach, with the tube lying in the oesophagus. Ventilation should be seen to cause a rise and fall of the chest, and a stethoscope should be used to confirm bilateral air entry. Improvement in the baby's colour should be seen after a few inflations of the lungs. The endotracheal tube should be held carefully in place, as it may easily enter one main bronchus or slip out of the trachea. It may be steadied against the corner of the baby's mouth during ventilation. Once the baby begins to breathe, he may be allowed to breathe oxygen via his endotracheal tube, without artificial ventilation, for a few breaths before extubation.

Intubation is a vital, life-saving skill, and must be learnt by clinical experience, and once learnt, the skill must be maintained. A stillborn baby provides a good model for initial attempts, and various artificial models are also available. Midwives may not always be encouraged to acquire this skill, but if they are likely to find themselves in a situation without other skilled assistance, they should equip themselves to carry out the procedure competently and with confidence.

If the heart rate remains below 60 despite the establishing of IPPV by mask or endotracheal tube for 20–30 seconds, cardiac massage may be necessary (unnecessary cardiac massage is dangerous). The hands should be placed around the baby's chest, with the fingers overlapping at the back and the thumbs together in front. The chest is then gently compressed from front to back, using the thumbs and moving them about 2 cm in and out, at a rate of 100–120/minute. The amount of compression is more easily controlled when this method is used. After every 3–4 compressions, the lungs should be inflated.

In an emergency situation where resuscitation equipment is not readily available, mouth-to-mouth resuscitation, though crude, may be life-saving. Here the importance of not overinflating the lungs must be reiterated. The operator fills her cheeks with air (or oxygen if available), and without making any expiratory effort of her own, covers the baby's nose and mouth with her mouth and gently puffs air in. Again, a rate of about 40 per minute is ideal.

The problem of how long resuscitative attempts should continue is a vexed question to which there is no definite answer. Prolonged resuscitation of a severely depressed baby has seen remarkably good results in some cases. However, such efforts will also present some parents with a severely handicapped child for many years. TSR — Time to Sustained Respiration — is considered an important factor in assessing the baby's progress and the success of resuscitation. Ideally, this should occur within one minute of birth, and generally speaking, the longer the TSR, the worse the prognosis, though most severely asphyxiated infants, if resuscitated well, will survive intact.

Failure to stimulate cardiac function adequately will obviously render all other measures ineffective, and probably most paediatricians would consider that 15 minutes or more of extreme bradycardia without sign of improvement would be incompatible with a reasonable quality of life. Causes of depression other than intra-partum hypoxia or drug-induced depression would be considered in such circumstances. These would include a misplaced endotracheal tube, congenital abnormality such as diaphragmatic hernia, intracranial haemorrhage (as in tentorial tear) and other birth injuries.

Successful resuscitation gives the following picture:
increased heart rate
improved blood pressure
colour improving from pale or blue to pink
spontaneous gasps, leading to normal respiration
presence of spinal reflexes
improved muscle tone

Prompt and appropriate resuscitation of the baby is clearly an essential part of obstetric services, and every midwife must be able to provide this facility whenever necessary.

## SUGGESTED FURTHER READING

Bonica, J. J. (1972) *Obstetric Analgesia and Anaesthesia.* Berlin: Springer-Verlag.

Chiswick, M. L. (1978) *Neonatal Medicine,* 1st edn. London: Update Publications.

Corke, B. C. (1977) Neurobehavioural responses of the newborn: the effect of different forms of maternal analgesia. *Anaesthesia* 32:539.

Keay, A. J. and Morgan, D. M. (1978) *Craig's Care of the Newly Born Infant,* 6th edn. Edinburgh: Churchill Livingstone.

Kelnar, C. J. H. and Harvey, D. (1981) *The Sick Newborn Baby.* London: Baillière Tindall.

Klaus, M. H. and Fanaroff, A. A. (1979) *Care of the High-Risk Neonate.* W. B. Saunders.

Moir, D. D. (1980) *Obstetric Anaesthesia and Analgesia,* 2nd edn. London: Baillière Tindall.

Sweet, B. R. (1982) *Mayes' Midwifery — A Textbook for Midwives,* 1st edn. London: Baillière Tindall.

# Index

Acetylcholine, 36
Acetylcholinesterase, 36
Acid aspiration, *see* Mendelŝon's
  syndrome
Acidosis, 47, 49, 73, 91
  reversal, 94
'Active birth', 6, 103
Adrenaline, 43, 72, 122, 130
Airways, 19, 85
  neonatal clearance, 158–159
Albumin, salt-poor, 93
Alcuronium, 36, 58
Alloferin, 36
Alphaloxone, 30–31
Althesin, 30–31
Amethocaine, 43, 146
Amide group, local anaesthetics,
  40–41
Anaesthesia
  and caesarean section, 56–59
  definition, 28
  drugs, 26–44
  nursing during, 66–73
  obstetric, problems, 83–95
    aortocaval occlusion, 86–87
    blood loss, 90–94
    difficult intubation, 87–90
    Mendelson's syndrome, 83–86
  obstetric, requirements, 52–55
  stages, 26–27
Analgesia

definition, 28
epidural, 6, 47, 123–143, 145
  inadequate or unilateral, 133
  inhalational, 4–5, 103, 114–122
  obstetric, 96–104
  other regional blocks, 144–150
  spinal, 144–148
  stage of anaesthesia, 26
Analgesics, *see under* Drugs, *also
  specific analgesics*, e.g. Morphine
Antacids, 56, 64
Antagonists, opiate, 38–39, 109
Ante-natal preparation, 101–102
Anti-emetics, 58
Anxiolysis, 29
Aortocaval occlusion, 46, 54
  cause, prevention, treatment,
    86–87
Apgar scores, 152, 153, 154
Apnoea, 152–154
Arterial
  blood gas analysis, 73
  occlusion, 80
  pressure monitoring, 78–79
Aspirin, 39
Assessment at birth, 152, 153
Assisting the anaesthetist, 67–70
Association of Obstetric
  Physiotherapists, 101–102
Atracurium, 36
Atropine, 36, 56, 59, 72

'Australia antigen positive', 23
Awareness, and lack of, 52–53, 81

Bain circuit, 14
Barbiturates, 110
Barbotage, 146
Beta-adrenergic agents, 111–112
Birth
  physiological changes, 154
  plan, 61
Blood
  clotting, 91
  fetal/maternal (F-M) ratios,
    47–48
  flow, placental, 49–50
  from 'banks', 92
  gas analysis, arterial, 73
  loss, 71, 90–94
  volume, 45–46, 90–91
'Bloody tap', 134
Bodok seals, 10–11
Bosun, 12
Boyles machine, 8–15
Bretylium, 72
Brietal, 30
Bupivacaine, 43, 130, 146

CSF (Cerebrospinal fluid), 128,
  134, 146–147
CVP (central venous pressure)
  lines, 76–78
Caesarean section, 52, 54, 56–59,
    88–89, 137–140
  induction of anaesthesia, 57
  maintenance, 58
  premedication, 56–57
  pre-oxygenation, 57, 88–89
  reversal, 59
Calcium gluconate, 72

Carbocaine, 146
Carbon dioxide, 32
  in blood, 59
Cardiac arrest, 71–73
  massage, external, 71–72
  principles of treatment, 73
Cardiff inhaler, 120, 121
Cardiff palliator, 107
Cardiovascular
  disease, and epidural analgesia,
    132
  system, 46, 91
    changes during labour, 46–47
Care, *see* Nursing
Catheters
  epidural, 128–129
  mounts, 18–19
  sterile suction, 156
Caudal epidural analgesia, 123–125
Central Midwives' Board, 4
Central venous pressure lines,
  76–78
Cerebrospinal fluid (CSF), 128,
  134, 146–147
Chloral hydrate, 110
Chloroform, 2, 34
Cimetidine, 56
Cinchocaine, 43, 146, 147
Circuits, Boyles machines, 13–14
Clotting
  blood, 91
  specific factors, 93
Coagulation abnormalities, 132
Cocaine, 1–2, 3, 43
Colour coding, 9
Complications, 78, 80, 133–135
'Crash induction', definition, 28
Cricoid pressure, 67–70
Curare, 1, 2, 5, 35, 58
Cyclopropane, 32

DIC (disseminated intravascular coagulation), 91
D-Tubocurarine, 35
Delirium stage, 26
Demerol, 106–108
Depolarization, 34, 41
Depolarizing relaxants, 35
Depressed infants, 152–154
Depression, infant, minimal, 53–54
Dextrans, 93
Diabetes mellitus, 131
Diamorphine, 37, 108
Diazepam, 110
Dichloralphenazone, 110
Diffusion, placental, 48–49
Disseminated intravascular coagulation (DIC), 91
Drugs
  in anaesthesia, 26–44
    basic principles and definitions, 26–29
    induction agents, 29–31
    local anaesthetic agents, 39–44
    maintenance agents, 31–34
    muscle relaxants, 34–37
    narcotics and analgesics, 37–39
    premedication, 29
  and placental blood flow, 49–50
  diffusion, 48–49
  emergency, 72–73
  in epidural analgesia, 130–131
  in labour, 105–113
    acting on uterus, 110–112
    parenteral narcotics, 105–110
    rules and regulations, 105–106
  *see also specific drugs, e.g.* Thiopentone
Dural tap, 134

Edrophonium, 37
Emergencies during anaesthesia, 70–73
Emergency oxygen flush, 12
Emotril automatic inhaler, 119, 120, 121
Endorphins, 98
Endotracheal
  extubation, 73
  intubation, 4, 52–53, 57
    difficulty with, 70, 87–90
    equipment, 15–19
    neonatal, 160
Enflurane, 33, 58
Enkephalins, 99
Entonox, 6, 115–119
Epidural analgesia, 6, 47, 123–143
  anatomy, 123
  and caesarean section, 137–140
  care following delivery, 141–142
  caudal, 123–125
  complications, 133–135
  contra-indications to, 132–133
  drugs, 130–131
  epidural blood patch, 136–137
  equipment, 126–128
  indications for, 131–132
  management of second stage of labour, 140–141
  nursing reponsibilities, 140
  post-partum discomforts and problems, 135–136
  preparation of patient, 125–126
  procedure, 128–130
  'topping up', 142–143
Epontol, 31
Equipment, 4–5, 8–25
  arterial lines, 79
  Boyles machine, 8–15

preparation, 64
central venous pressure lines,
76–77
'difficult intubation', 90
Entonox, 116–118
for endotracheal intubation,
15–19
preparation, 65–66
for epidural analgesia, 126–128
for resuscitating newborn,
155–158
for spinal analgesia, 145
Lucy Baldwin apparatus,
117–118
operating table, 23–25
theatre hazards, 22–23
ventilators, 21–22
Ergometrine, 58, 111
Esters, local anaesthetics, 40–41
Ether, 2, 34
Ethrane, 33
Etomidate, 31
Excitement stage, 26
Explosion risks, 22–23
Extradural analgesia, *see*
Epidural analgesia

FFP (fresh frozen plasma), 92
F/M(fetal/maternal) blood ratios,
47–48
Face masks, 14–15, 156
Fazadinium (Fazadon), 36
Fentanyl, 37, 38
Fentazin, 110
Fetus, drug effects on, 50
Fibrinogen, 93
Fire risks, 22–23
Flaxedil, 36
Fluids
clear, 94

replacement therapy, 91–94
Fluothane, 33
Fortral, 39, 108
Fresh frozen plasma (FFP), 92

Gallamine, 36
Gas and air, 4
Gases, 31–32
cylinders, 11–13
changing, 11–12
in Boyles machines, 8–11
*see also specific gases*, e.g. Nitrous
oxide
Gate control theory, 98
Guedel airway, 19
Glycopyrrolate, 57

HPPF (human plasma protein
fraction), 92–93
Haemaccel, 93
Haemorrhage, 71, 90–94
Halothane, 6, 33, 58, 112
Hazards, operating theatre, 22–23
Head harness, 20
Hearing, and anaesthesia, 53
Heroin, 37
History, 1–7
Human plasma protein fraction
(HPPF), 92–93
Hyoscine, 56
Hyperventilation, 45
Hypnomidate, 31
Hypnosis, 103
Hypnotics, 103, 110
definition, 28
Hypoglycaemia, 48–49
Hypotension, 71, 133
Hypoxia, 54, 71, 73, 152–154

I-D (induction-delivery) interval, 54

Identity checks, 64, 66
Induction agents, 29–31, 54
  and caesarean section, 57
Infant depression, 152–154
  minimal, 53–54
Inhalational analgesia, 4–5, 103,
  114–122
  methoxyflurane, 120–122
  nitrous oxide, 115–119
  trichloroethylene, 119–120
Intensive care, 75–80
Intraval, 30
IPPV (intermittent positive
  pressure ventilation)
  adult, 21
  neonatal, 159–160
Isoprenaline, 72

Ketalar, 31
Ketamine, 31
Ketosis, 47, 49, 73, 91
  reversal, 94

Labour
  drugs, 105–113
  premature, 132
  second stage management,
    140–141
Laryngoscopes, 16–17, 155
Legal requirements, 105–106,
  114–115
Lethidrone, 38, 109, 157
Levallorphan, 38, 109, 157
Lidocaine, 43, 72
Lignocaine, 42, 43, 130, 146, 147
Local anaesthetics, 39–44, 102
Lorfan, 38, 109, 157
Lucy Baldwin apparatus, 4–5,
  117–118
Lungs, neonatal, 154, 159–160

Macintosh laryngoscope, 16
Magill
  circuit, 13
  forceps, 19, 20
  laryngoscope, 17
Maintenance agents, 31–34, 54
  caesarean section, 58
Malpresentation, 131
Marcain, 43, 130
Masks, face, 14–15, 156
Medicines Act, and Order, 105
Medullary paralysis, 27
Mendelson's syndrome, 59, 67,
  83–86
  causes, 83–84
  prevention, 52, 84–85
  treatment, 85–86
Meperidine, 106–108
Mepivacaine, 146
Metabolic acidosis, 47, 49, 73, 91
  reversal, 94
Methohexitone, 30
Methoxyflurane, 6, 33–34,
  120–122
Metoclopramide, 85
Minnitt's apparatus, 4
Mist. magnesium trisilicate, 56, 84
Misuse of Drugs Act, and
  Regulations, 105
Monitoring during recovery, 75
Morphine, 4, 37, 108
Mouth gags and props, 19–20
Mouth-to-mouth resuscitation, 72,
  161
Multiple pregnancy, 131
Muscle relaxants, 5, 34–37, 54
Myometrium–delivery interval, 54

Nalorphine, 38, 109, 157
Naloxone (Narcan), 39, 109, 157

Narcotics, 37–39
  antagonists, 38–39, 109
  definition, 28
  parenteral, 105–110
  *see also specific narcotics*, e.g.
    Pethidine
National Childbirth Trust, 101
Neonatal resuscitation equipment,
  155–158
Neostigmine, 36, 59
Nerves, *see* Pain pathways
Neurobehavioural tests, 50
Neuroleptanaesthesia, definition,
  28
Neurological disease, and epidural
  analgesia, 133
Neuromuscular transmission, 34,
  41
Nitrous oxide, 2, 3, 4, 31, 58
  and oxygen, 115–119
Non-depolarizing relaxants, 35–37
Nupercaine, 43, 146, 147
Nursing
  care plan, 61, 62
  process, 60–62
  responsibilities, 60–82, 140–142
    during anaesthesia, 66–73
    patient requiring intensive
      care, 75–80
    patient on ventilator, 80–82
    pre-operative period, 62–66
    recovery period, 74–75

Obstetric analgesia, 96–104
  pain pathways, 96–99
  in labour, 99–100
  relief, 101–103
Occipitoposterior position, 131
Omnopon, 38
Operating tables, 23–25

Operidine, 37, 38
Opiates, 37–38, 102, 106–108
  antagonists, 38–39, 109
  endogenous, 98–99
  and epidural analgesia, 130–131
    139
  post caesarean delivery, 58
Opium, 2
Oxford needle, 148, 149
Oxygen, 32, 58
  and nitrous oxide, 115–119
Oxygenation, 49
Oxytocin, 110–111
Oxytoxics, 58, 110–111

PABA (para-aminobenzoic acid),
  41
PEEP (Positive End Expiratory
  Pressure), 21, 81
Packed cells, 92
Pain pathways, 96–99
  in labour, 99–100
Pain relief, 101–103
Pancuronium, 36, 58
Papaveretum, 38
Para-aminobenzoic acid, 41
Paracervical block, 148–149
Paracetamol, 39
Parenteral narcotics, 105–110
Patients
  intensive care, 75–80
  monitoring, 75
  positioning during anaesthesia,
    66–67
  positioning during recovery,
    74–75
  preparation, 62–64
    for epidural analgesia, 125–126
  reception, 66
  unconscious, care of, 74–75

on ventilator, 80–81
Pavulon, 36
Pentazocine, 39, 108
Penthrane, 33–34, 120–122
Pentothal, 30
Peridural analgesia, *see*
  Epidural analgesia
Peripheral vasodilation, 94
Perphenazine, 110
Pethidine, 5, 37, 50, 106–108
Pethilorfan, 5, 109
Pharmacology
  of local anaesthetics, 40
  and physiology, 45–51
Phenergan, 109
Phenobarbitone, 47
Phenoperidine, 37, 38
Physical preparation, 63–64
  for epidural analgesia, 125–126
Physiology
  changes in neonates, 154
  and pharmacology, 45–51
    physiology in pregnancy,
      45–47
    placental transfer, 47–50
Physostigmine, 37
Placental transfer, 47–50
  barrier, 47–49
  blood flow, 49–50
Plasma expanders/substitutes, 93
Platelets, 93
Pneumothorax, 78
Pontocaine, 43, 146
Positioning, 66–67, 74
  'active birth', 103
Positive End Expiratory Pressure
  (PEEP), 21, 81
Pre-eclampsia, 131
Premedication, 29
  for caesarean section, 56–57

Pre-operative nursing, 62–66
Pre-oxygenation, for caesarean
  section, 57
Problems
  identification, 60–62
  in obstetric anaesthesia, 83–95
Procaine, 3, 4, 42
Prochlorperazine, 110
Promazine, 109
Promethazine, 109
Propanidid, 31
Prostaglandins, 39, 98, 111
  inhibition, 112
Prostigmine, 36
Protein binding, 49
Pseudocholinesterase, 35, 41
Psychological preparation, 62–63,
  101–102
Psychoprophylaxis, 5
Pudendal block, 149
Pyridostigmine, 37

Ranitidine, 56
Recovery period nursing, 74–75
  care of unconscious patient,
    74–75
  observation and monitoring, 75
Relaxants, 34–37, 54
Renal system, 46
Requirements in obstetric
  anaesthesia, 52–55
  lack of maternal awareness,
    52–53
  minimal depression of infant,
    53–54
  prevention of Mendelson's
    syndrome, 52
Respiratory distress syndrome,
  47
Respiratory system, changes

in pregnancy, 45
Responsibilities, nursing, 60–82
140–142
Resuscitaire, 155–158
Resuscitation of neonates, 151–162
anticipating need, 151–152
assessment, 152
depressed infant, 152–154
equipment, 155–158
physiological changes at birth, 154
principles, 158–162
Reversal agents, 36
caesarean section, 59
Ritodrine, 112
Robinul, 57

Saddle block, 147
Salbutamol, 112
Scoline, 35, 57, 58
Scopolamine, 4
Sedatives, definition, 28
Sellick's manoeuvre, 69–70
Sensory tracts, *see* Pain pathways
Serum hepatitis, 23
'Silver swaddlers', 156
Sodium bicarbonate, 72, 157
Sodium citrate, 56, 84
Sparine, 109
Specific clotting factors, 93
Spinal
anaesthesia, 144–148
blocks, in obstetrics, 147–148
drugs, 130–131
headache, 134, 144
Stages of anaesthesia, 26–27
Stemetil, 110
Steroids, 47

Subarachnoid block, *see*
Spinal anaesthesia
Sublimaze, 37, 38
Supine hypotensive syndrome, *see*
Aortacaval occlusion
Surgical anaesthesia, 26–27
Suxamethonium, 35, 57, 58
Syntocinon, 58
Syntometrine, 111

Tecota inhaler, 119, 120, 121
Teeth, 64
Tensilon, 37
Terminology, 28–29
Tetracaine, 43, 146
Thiopentone, 30, 57
Throat spray, 20
Thrombo-phlebitis, 78
Tocolytics, 111–112
'Topping-up' epidural blocks, 141, 142–143
'Total spinal', 134-135
Toxicity, local anaesthetics, 41-42, 134
Tracheotomy, 71
Tracrium, 36
Tranquillizers, 103, 109–110
definition, 29
Trichloroethylene, 5, 33, 58, 119–120
Trichloryl (Trichlofos), 110
Trilene, 33, 58, 119–120
TSR (time to sustained respiration), 161
Tubarine, 35
Tuohy needle, 127-129
'Twilight sleep', 4

U-D(Myometrium-delivery)
interval, 54
Unconscious patient care, 74
United Kingdom Central Council
for Nursing, Midwifery & Health
Visiting, 105–106, 114–115, 142
Uterus
drugs, 110–112
incoordinate action, 132
scarred, 132–133

Vagal blockade, 29

Valves, reducing, 8, 10
Vaporizers, 12–13
Ventilators
care of patients, 80–81
equipment, 21–22
Volatile agents, 32–34

Welldorm, 110

Xylocaine, 43

Yutopar, 112